MENOPOCALYPSE

AMANDA THEBE

MENOPO

CALYPSE

How I Learned to Thrive During Menopause and How You Can Too

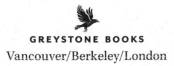

GREYSTONE BOOKS

Vancouver/Berkeley/London

Greystone Books Ltd.
greystonebooks.com

Cataloguing data available from Library and Archives Canada
ISBN 978-1-77164-760-1 (pbk.)
ISBN 978-1-77164-761-8 (epub)

Editing by Nancy Flight
Copyediting by Jess Shulman
Proofreading by Jennifer Stewart
Cover design by Nayeli Jimenez
Text design by Fiona Siu
Cover photograph by Audra Oden
Photographs by Alicia Merrifield

Printed and bound in Canada on FSC° certified paper at Friesens.
The FSC° label means that materials used for the product have
been responsibly sourced.

The advice in this book has been carefully considered and checked by the
author and publisher. It should not, however, be regarded as a substitute for
medical advice. We recommend talking to your doctor before starting any
new exercise routine.

Greystone Books thanks the Canada Council for the Arts, the British
Columbia Arts Council, the Province of British Columbia through the Book
Publishing Tax Credit, and the Government of Canada for supporting our
publishing activities.

Canadä

    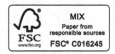

BRITISH COLUMBIA

BRITISH COLUMBIA ARTS COUNCIL
An agency of the Province of British Columbia

Canada Council   Conseil des arts
for the Arts   du Canada

FSC
www.fsc.org

MIX
Paper from
responsible sources
FSC° C016245

Greystone Books gratefully acknowledges the xʷməθkʷəy̓əm (Musqueam),
Sḵwx̱wú7mesh (Squamish), and səlilwətaɬ (Tsleil-Waututh) peoples on
whose land our Vancouver head office is located.

CONTENTS

HOW I BECAME A MENOPAUSE WARRIOR

THE CHINESE CALL it "a woman's second spring." Westerners call it "the change." I call it "menopocalypse." Yes, I am talking about menopause.

My journey into the unknown started with perimenopause and culminated in my current postmenopausal state. And what a journey it has been! I consider it one of the toughest ordeals of my life, especially since I have always been so healthy and physically fit.

As a child growing up in northeast England, I started doing karate at age eleven and have been motivated to exercise and eat well ever since. As I got older, fitness remained a passion, and I spent my time outside of my job at IBM working to become a personal trainer.

After meeting my husband and immigrating to North America, I embarked on a new career in graphic design but maintained my passion for fitness, coaching friends at the local YMCA or training mums in the schoolyard. In 2013, I finally decided to leave my design business to start my own fitness company, Fit n' Chips, and have not looked back since.

My business thrived. I had the most amazing clients, and they inspired me to be a better coach and person. I am embarrassed to recall how dismissive I used to be of women who complained about menopause and its symptoms. I encouraged them to just push through their discomfort and work harder. I mean, how awful could "the change" be? There was little to no information available for a personal trainer working with menopausal women, and having not yet experienced menopause myself, I just could not relate. Today I eat humble pie. As soon as the shit hit the fan for me, everything they had told me made sense, and those early discussions have helped me immensely with my research. (P.S. I'm sorry!)

Entering my forties felt like a breeze. I was fit and healthy and in better condition both physically and mentally than I had been in my twenties. I felt awesome and thought I looked awesome, too. I was clearly doing something right, and I could see that it was inspiring other women to get strong, look after themselves, and thrive in their forties as well. Life was good. I was living the dream!

Then I turned forty-three.

Something happened that changed everything I knew about my body and my health. It started after one of my bi-weekly boxing classes, where I worked exceptionally hard, punching a huge heavy bag with all my might. I loved that class (it reminded me of my old karate days), but that afternoon I had to go home and lie down. I assumed I had just pushed a little too hard in the class. You know that feeling when you're on a high after an epic workout but afterward are so spent that all you want to do is sleep? That was me.

But after I lay down, I couldn't get back up again. It felt like my bed was spinning. I began to feel nauseous, and my whole equilibrium shifted. I realized I was experiencing some kind of vertigo, and I was literally seeing stars.

This condition lasted for two days and was completely debilitating. After it subsided I just assumed it had been some sort of virus. I quickly got back to normal, but a few days later it hit me again, and then again, and again.

I had no idea what was happening to me. My head would feel like it was being squeezed in a vise, and then I'd experience extreme nausea and vomiting. I couldn't walk without falling over, so I crawled around on my hands and knees. It was just horrid.

Each of these episodes would last three to five days, and they happened almost every week, leaving me utterly exhausted. It was a hellish time for me, as my new business had just started to flourish and I was eager to invest time and energy in it. Yet most of the time I felt so unwell I could barely even make myself a cup of tea. I remember reading a bedtime story to my six-year-old, just wishing it to be over so I could hit the sack—at seven o'clock! I don't remember ever feeling that tired before or since, even when the children were newborns.

I eventually went to see my doctor, leading to many visits to neurologists and ENTs (ear, nose, and throat specialists). I underwent dozens of tests, including an MRI, a CT scan, balance testing in which vertigo was induced, and many more. For more than eighteen months I went back and forth to the hospital. One time I landed in the emergency room because I felt so unwell. All of the tests came back inconclusive. Without any answers, I spiraled into despair. The doctors recognized that something was clearly wrong with me: I felt like shit and I looked like shit, but none of them—*none of them*—could help me. What was happening to me?

After almost two years of struggling with these symptoms, I couldn't remember what it was like to feel good. I consider myself to be a hardy person; I very rarely get sick, and when I do, I tend to handle it quite well. Even that ability was compromised now.

Inevitably this had an impact on my emotional well-being. I started to withdraw from social events, which was completely out of character for me—I love a good party. Some days, after coaching my clients, I would drive straight home, collapse onto the sofa, and just stare into space, unable to move and unable to care. The only thing that stopped me from sitting there into the night was that I had to collect my children from school.

On the other side of this despair was a side to my character that really scared me. It was like a switch would flip, and I would suddenly fly into a hysterical rage. I would shout, scream, and cry like a wild banshee. I didn't even recognize myself, my head spinning like something out of *The Exorcist*. I still get tears in my eyes thinking of how scared my own kids were of me, wondering if I was going to be nice Mam or crazy-bitch-from-hell Mam that day. No mother wants her children to be scared of her; mine were walking around on eggshells.

They say you get to a certain point along the road where you have no choice but to take action. One night, when I was feeling particularly low, I attacked my husband out of the blue with a list of all the things I didn't like about him.

It was horrible. I was horrible. He didn't stand a chance against the angry volley of verbal abuse I was throwing at him. Exhausted and worried for our marriage, he asked if we were going to be okay. He didn't want the marriage to break down and would do anything to help me, to help us.

The realization hit me then. All of the wretched things I had just told him I hated were actually things I admired about him (my hubby was born without tact, yet one of the things I love about him most is that he cannot lie. If you want to know the harsh truth, he'll give it to you! I wish I could be more like that). I had a moment of intense clarity where I saw that my marriage was (and still is) a good, strong marriage. I loved my husband and children, we were financially secure, my business was thriving, I had lots of amazing friends and a good support network— so why was I so unhappy? I knew in that moment that I needed to get help and to start getting answers.

In the end it was a routine appointment with my gynecologist that saved my soul and my marriage, and definitely my sanity. After two years of visits to other specialists, I went in for my regular well-woman examination. I usually hate those appointments, where the doctor rushes through the fifteen minutes allotted to you with little empathy and makes it seem almost impossible to ask the questions that are bothering you. I always feel like a bloody nuisance and then struggle to find the right words to describe exactly how I'm feeling.

This time, though, was different. As the appointment was ending, my doctor stopped, looked me straight in the eye, and saw that something wasn't right.

"Are you okay?" he asked.

"No, I'm not!"

The tears started and wouldn't stop. All it took was for him to ask me if I was okay and then to actually listen to me. Of course he'd seen this all before, but I had no idea what was happening to my mind or my body, who I was becoming, and where the real me had gone.

He immediately recognized what I was experiencing: perimenopause. All of the symptoms that had been dragging me down were very real perimenopausal symptoms. I was suffering from chronic depression, caused in part by my fluctuating estrogen levels, which was something he could help me with. My vertigo, nausea, and balance issues were all the result of migraine with aura, another known and treatable symptom of perimenopause.

I am not one of those people who head to Google to fill themselves with fear about all the dreadful things that could be wrong with them; in fact, I tend to use Google as a way to rule out illnesses. But I had been starting to think that something was seriously wrong with me, so when I finally found out what was really happening, I was flooded with relief. Even though my symptoms were horrible and life-altering, it was reassuring to know that they were part of a normal process that my body had to go through and was well-equipped for—though it might need some assistance. My doctor told me of treatments and protocols I could follow to start gaining control again. At last I had an answer. At last I could start the process of feeling better.

Now I just needed to understand what the hell perimenopause was! My symptoms over those past two years had included depression, erratic mood swings, migraines with aura, fatigue, short-term memory loss, loss of motor skills, and incontinence (yep, that too!), and they could all be explained by my fluctuating hormones. I'm not going to lie, I was pissed off that I had endured over a year and a half of tests and visits to ENTs and neurologists, and for some reason they couldn't see the bloody obvious staring them in the face. Yet it took just five minutes with my gynecologist to identify what was happening. What a relief it was to finally know that I wasn't going crazy, that this was an actual thing that had a name. And so began my journey to peel back the layers of what perimenopause really is and to share that information with other women out there.

The biggest lesson was that I had to advocate for myself and my health. I had to keep asking questions and pushing for answers, despite constantly being told there was no conclusive reason that I felt the way I did. I was living in Canada, a country where I had easy access to a medical team—and yet I felt that team had failed me.

I can't highlight this enough: women are still experiencing dismissive medical care, leaving us feeling all sorts of crazy, simply because our symptoms aren't readily recognized. Had I known that these were symptoms of perimenopause, I could have gone to my appointments armed with this information and asked for help. In hindsight, I realized that I had in fact started feeling perimenopausal not long after the birth of my second child. Around the age of thirty-eight, my periods had started to change, and so did my PMS. I'd often been hit with really bad fatigue, and my immunity to colds and bugs was compromised, so I often felt run-down.

Why didn't I have this information? It seems so obvious to me now that had I known, I could have coped with my situation much better.

Women are given very little information about menopause. It isn't taught in schools, GPs don't get training in menopause management, it's not discussed in the work-place, and even among friends it's rarely discussed openly.

When I frantically tried to find information online, it quickly became apparent that the pickings were slim. Information on websites felt dumbed down to include only hot flashes and a few mood swings. The reality can be so very different. Historically, women have been hugely underrepresented in research; it appears we are too dif-ficult to study, you know, because we have periods and complicated hormones.

In her 2018 book *Doing Harm: The Truth About How Bad Medicine and Lazy Science Leave Women Dismissed, Mis-diagnosed, and Sick*, Maya Dusenbery discusses a study from the early sixties. "Observing that women tended to have lower rates of heart disease until their estrogen levels dropped after menopause, researchers conducted the first trial to look at whether supplementation with the hormone was an effective preventive treatment. The study enrolled 8,341 men and no women." Today women may be getting more of the attention they deserve: as recently as 2016, the National Institutes of Health deemed that any research it funds must include female animals, removing the male bias in scientific studies. Despite this, there is still much more research needed for women in menopause.

What else did I learn? That I was not taking the fight lying down, that I was taking charge of my life again by being proactive and recognizing that nutrition, exercise, recovery, relaxation, and stress reduction were key to making this period of my life manageable. A strength and metabolically challenging fitness program that focused on building lean muscle and keeping my metabolism revved up was imperative. On the flip side, prioritizing recovery and relaxation was also critical, so that my body could heal. Limiting shitty foods laden with added sugar and refined within an inch of their lives helped keep my migraines at bay and my moods lifted—bingeing on overly processed foods with ingredients I couldn't pronounce (which I seemed to crave more than ever in my life) made me hit rock bottom. Alcohol became my enemy (and trust me—taking away a gin and tonic from a northern lass is not a pretty sight); I simply could not tolerate it without dire side effects. (Side note: I'm really hoping to get that resilience back, as I can't wait to get a little tipsy again!)

As well as all of the above, I found that for the first time in my life, I needed to take time each day for me. That was something I had never done, but finding the time each day to read, nap, knit, go for a walk, or do anything that pressed my reset button became vitally important.

And finally, I started talking—talking about my symptoms to anybody and everybody. And I haven't stopped. I don't care if it makes them roll their eyes in boredom. I know that women want and deserve to be heard. We're tired of being ignored, misunderstood, and belittled. We're sick of feeling invisible. If I can do anything with this book, I want to change that whole dynamic. I am happy to put my vagina on the line for this cause.

My experience is what led me to write this book. Most people don't realize that perimenopause (or menopause transition) can start affecting women in their late thirties or early forties. Perimenopause is the phase when most symptoms appear, and they can last up to ten years. Women are considered menopausal at the point in time that it has been twelve consecutive months since their last period ended. And that's just the beginning, baby! After that day, a woman is postmenopausal, and we are in fact postmenopausal till death do us part. A woman can spend more than a third of her life in menopause—from perimenopause to postmenopause—and with women's average life expectancy hovering around eighty-one in North America, that's a bloody long time.

Whether you are a woman heading toward menopause, the husband/partner or son/daughter of a woman, or a trainer, counselor, teacher, coach, or employer who has female clients, students, or employees in their late thirties or beyond, you should get familiar with the impact that menopause can have on a woman. It's not fun, it's not sexy, and it usually makes people roll their eyes and want to walk in the other direction. But it's essential that we all become less embarrassed to talk about it and remove the shame and taboo that is associated with the unmentionable M-word.

I am now in the stage called postmenopause, as I haven't had a period for more than a year. I feel now that I have clarity about what has passed and what to expect next, yet one of the most frustrating things that I hear from women is that they have no idea what the hell is happening. Our mothers either told us nothing or minimized their experiences; it's just the way it was done in their generation. Women basically just got on with it and suffered in silence. But that's not me. I have a very loud voice, and I don't mind using it. I am ready to clear up confusion, dispel a few myths, and throw some truth bombs your way.

Using my experience and knowledge, as well as expert advice, I was eventually able to manage my symptoms and regain a normal life. This had a positive effect on my marriage and my family because, yeah, nice Mammy is back again!

What this book is and what it is not:

- This is a book to help you manage the things you can control so that you can cope with the ups and downs of menopause.

  › Part 1 of the book might seem full of doom and gloom; it's where I lay out all the shitty stuff happening. Persevere until Part 2.

  › Part 2 is where we get deep and dirty into solution-driven actions you can take today.

- This book is not a medical text. I have written it using the knowledge I have gained as a personal trainer and nutrition coach and from interviews with medical experts in the field of menopause management.

- This book is not a replacement for your chosen medical therapy.

Use this book as a companion to your work with your medical team. Any time you're having menopausal symptoms, I want you to reach for this book for guidance and support. I hope this book will be your new best friend.

PART ONE

THE REALITY

— 1 —

DEFINING THE MONSTER

I REMEMBER THAT MEETING with my gynecologist so well. When he told me I was experiencing perimenopause, he followed up with, "Have you had any hot flashes yet?" What the hell? Hot flashes? I was only forty-four years old! I couldn't believe he was asking me that question. If you're like me, the info on your birth certificate doesn't compute with how you feel, so the idea of having a middle-aged-lady ailment like hot flashes seemed completely preposterous. I was way too young for that shit!

The truth is that you can start noticing changes associated with perimenopause in your thirties. They might be minor at first, but if you're already seeing menstrual changes and/or emotional disturbances, this could be the start for you. I would go a step further and say that if you think you're experiencing perimenopause, then chances are that you are.

WHAT THE FECK IS MENOPAUSE ANYWAY?

Despite the need for more research, there *is* a ton of science about menopause. It includes lots of strange scientific terms, descriptions of confusing hormonal interactions, and information that mere mortals like me struggle to understand—and I don't think we need to. Understanding just the basics of menopause can go a long way in helping you get the best out of your experience.

Let's start by defining exactly what menopause is. Menopause can be broken down into three distinct phases: perimenopause, menopause, and postmenopause.

PERIMENOPAUSE

Years before the cycle of my period became erratic, I realized that the way my body reacted to my upcoming monthly period was changing in ways that weren't common PMS symptoms. For example, the fatigue that would overwhelm me the week beforehand would lay me out cold. No matter how much sleep I got, I was still exhausted. My performance in my workouts suffered greatly at this time; I barely had the strength to lift my usual weights, and anything metabolically demanding was completely out of the question.

I also had the most bizarre symptoms. As my periods approached, I would get a cold and a sore throat, and I couldn't stop sneezing—I had an overall increased intolerance to allergies. In the past I had usually suffered few or no PMS symptoms, so I thought this had to be something else. But sure enough, I could feel those symptoms leaving me as soon as the blood started to flow. I was only thirty-eight, but I know now that this was the start of some hormonal changes and the beginning of perimenopause.

Perimenopause means the period before menopause. This is the time in a woman's life when her hormonal cycles start shifting, paving the way for the natural transition, and it's probably the most symptomatic phase of menopause. Perimenopause can start as early as age thirty-five and can last for eight to ten years. Women still have their period and can still get pregnant during perimenopause, but they might also start suffering from a number of symptoms, which we'll look at in this chapter.

By providing realistic expectations and knowledge about perimenopause, I hope that I can help women prepare for the onslaught and manage through it. This proactive, solution-based approach to health can make a world of difference.

MENOPAUSE

Menopause means the "end of monthly cycles."

Has it been twelve months since your last period? If so, on the day you hit that twelve-month point, you can officially say you've hit menopause. You can reach menopause any time during your forties or fifties; the average age in North America is currently fifty-one. At this point the ovaries completely cease producing the sex hormones estrogen and progesterone, and you have reached the end of your childbearing years.

Smokers have been shown to start menopause up to two years earlier than the average. Menopause can also be induced by some drugs, by surgical removal of the ovaries, or by ovary damage from radiation cancer treatment. Such cases are sometimes referred to as forced menopause. If a woman has to take drugs to suppress estrogen in her body—such as tamoxifen, which may be prescribed following cancer treatment—the symptoms of menopause can be much more severe.

Additionally, some women will experience primary menopause (meaning before the age of forty), sometimes referred to as primary ovarian insufficiency (POI). Approximately 1 in 1,000 women suffer from POI, yet they are often misdiagnosed, as there is very little awareness of the condition. Doctors don't always associate the loss of periods, hot flashes, vaginal dryness, and mood swings at such an early age with the onset of menopause. A POI diagnosis can be obtained by testing a woman's FSH (follicle-stimulating hormone) and estradiol levels.

Technically menopause is simply a snapshot in time, that one day in your life, before you move to the next stage, postmenopause. You don't get a marching band or fireworks when it happens. It's usually just a regular old day!

There are times throughout this book when I use the term "menopause" to refer to the whole journey from peri- to postmenopause. Most publications, organizations, and websites of any standing use the term this way. The North American Menopause Society (NAMS), for example, talks about menopause symptoms, the menopause journey, and the menopause experience when they're talking about the whole shebang.

POSTMENOPAUSE

Once a woman has reached menopause, she is then referred to as postmenopausal. This is when you might start to see a decrease in some of the symptoms of peri-menopause, but that doesn't mean your symptoms will completely disappear. I've had clients who were still experiencing hot flashes in their seventies. Postmenopause is also a time when other health concerns—such as osteoporosis, Alzheimer's, and heart disease—might appear as a result of the decreased estrogen and progesterone in the body.

Other physical symptoms seem to be more prevalent at this stage. Scientists have shown that reaching menopause can speed up cellular aging; women may get more wrinkles, gain more weight, and lose more hair. It can be a hard thing for women to come to terms with. Often women in postmenopause feel that they've been written off by society because they aren't living up to some ridiculous youthful standard.

But my experience shows me that this is a powerful time in a woman's life, and we need to harness its potential. I have found strength from the struggles I've overcome to get to this place, and I am grateful for what my body and mind can handle—that they are so resilient. This strength has transferred over to other aspects of my life, and I feel more empowered than ever to put myself first and strive for personal success.

I have also found it a great opportunity to change the narrative about what aging looks like. Ladies, we need to embrace our wrinkles; we are so much more than how we look. Going through menopause also gives us the power to care less about what people think of us. It's a time to embrace the Beth Ditto line, "I have no control over what other people think of me, but I have 100% control of what I think of myself."

It's liberating. I don't feel the pressure to
conform. To be 'nice.' I'm not defined by how I look.
I'm finally a person, rather than a girl or woman
judged on her appearance. I'm allowed to have
opinions again. Mostly, though, I like just not caring
nearly so much about what people think of me.

PAULA SHERIDAN, Menopausing So Hard member

I HAD NO idea about the three stages of menopause, and I
discovered I'd been relying on hearsay. There are so many
myths and misconceptions out there that it's worth spending some time explaining what menopause isn't.

MENOPAUSE BELIEFS

Belief: Your periods just stop. Then, after twelve months,
you are in menopause.

Truth: Even ten years ago, in my naiveté, I assumed that
when a woman went through menopause, she simply
stopped having her period and a joyous state of affairs
ensued, where you couldn't get pregnant anymore, you
stopped menstruating, you didn't have to buy tampons
anymore, and you never had to worry about those dreadful
monthly moods. When I speak to other women who have
not yet experienced perimenopause or menopause, this is
exactly what they think is going to happen. Unfortunately,
the truth for most women is that this is definitely not so.

It wasn't until I experienced perimenopause myself that I
realized something entirely different happens. Most women

will have disruptive menstrual timelines, with periods occurring outside the regular twenty-eight-day cycle. Their periods may be heavier or lighter than usual, and they may have no periods for months and then have multiple bleedings in one month. I was all over the place; I never knew when my period would come. I had one period that lasted six weeks. At times my period was so heavy it was like I was birthing an alien—I was sure I'd need an iron infusion. Then I would go for up to seven months without a period, only to be surprised one morning by an uninvited guest to my Queen V party. This uncertainty was devastating.

Your hormones are fluctuating all the time during perimenopause, and you have to roll with the punches. You just have to expect the unexpected, unless you're on birth control or hormone therapy (HT), which regulate your hormones to a certain degree (see Chapter 2: The Good, the Bad, and the Ugly of HT). There are a few glorious women (approximately 10 percent) who truly will sail through the menopause journey unscathed, and I hope they are rejoicing and sipping champers waiting for the rest of us to emerge on the other side. At any one time there are going to be more than thirty million women in perimenopause or reaching menopause in North America. I mean, seriously, can you even imagine what that hormonal soup looks like? Understanding and educating yourself about what might happen during this time can make the whole experience manageable.

Belief: Menopause makes your sex drive take a nosedive.

Truth: It might. It can. Mine did! My husband asked me if going through perimenopause was going to make me hornier. "I hope so" was my response, but unfortunately for me—and him—my desire tanked. In fact, it was hard to call it low libido when I felt completely removed from the idea of having sex at all. It was more like I had an apathy toward sex—apart from those rare occasions when I became a raging nymphomaniac, climbing the walls in frustration if I didn't get laid immediately (okay, this happened twice, but still it did happen).

Truthfully, the answer is "it depends." Most women see their libido drop to the point that they are miserable (according to the WHO, about 68 to 86 percent of menopausal women experience sexual dysfunction), but for a minority of women it's business as usual. Vaginal atrophy and dryness, and in some cases incontinence, can make sex more uncomfortable and less desirable. Chapter 4 discusses this topic in more detail.

Belief: Menopause makes you fat.

Truth: Most menopausal women are overweight. I know you do not want to hear that, but the research shows this to be true. A study from the National Health and Nutrition Examination Survey (NHANES) data found that 68 percent of women aged forty to fifty-nine were classified as "overweight" or "affected by obesity." This number increased to 78.3 percent for women over sixty, who are most likely postmenopausal. Now to be clear, this isn't all menopause's fault, but the age range is significant, as we know this is when the majority of women will go through the stages of menopause.

Most women report gaining up to five pounds during their menopause journey; I probably gained closer to ten.

In fact, the report shows that 20 percent of women studied gained ten pounds or more.

But don't despair; you need to know why weight gain happens before you freak out. I am going to share the cold hard truth about weight gain with you and the solutions that will help you avoid becoming one of those statistics.

Belief: The only symptom you get with menopause is hot flashes—they aren't so bad, are they?

Truth: Bullshit. I had symptoms practically falling out of my vagina.

Belief: I'm too young for menopause.

Truth: Really, you think so? You think it's just for old ladies way past their prime, not fresh and vibrant like you? Many women are confused about when perimenopause starts, and I don't blame them. I've had women in their late forties believing it wasn't even possible they were in perimenopause, because they had this idea that it would happen sometime in their fifties or later. That's where education and understanding really help. Let's get deep and dirty into hormones.

MEET THE HORMONES

To review, when you're going through menopause, the sex hormones in your ovaries are going to stop coming out to play. They're outta here, baby, so you might as well meet these fleeting lovelies and see the type of destruction they leave in their wake.

ESTROGEN: YOUR HAPPY HORMONE

The main player in the menopause game, estrogen, is responsible for so many functions in the body (see below) that when its levels start to diminish, the symptoms can present themselves in numerous ways. As you go through perimenopause, your estrogen starts to decline, but not in a linear fashion; rather it fluctuates up and down, which can lead to a myriad of symptoms. Its erratic nature during perimenopause can leave women feeling as though they've been hit by a truck that's then reversed and run them over again for good measure. When you understand how powerful estrogen is, you can more easily understand what is happening to you. Losing such an important aid to your body can have effects that have typically been ridiculously understated.

Estrogen is produced mainly in the ovaries but also in small amounts in the adrenal glands and fat cells.

Roles of estrogen in your body:

- Promotes the growth and health of the female reproductive organs

- Keeps the vagina moisturized, elastic (stretchy), and well supplied with blood

- Helps to form serotonin (a mood enhancer), saving you and those in close proximity to you from irritability and anxiety; there are estrogen receptors all over the brain

- Along with vitamin D and calcium, helps with bone formation

- Plays a role in the health of other systems in the body, including the heart, the brain, hair, skin, and breasts, as well as a role during pregnancy

- Is an anabolic (meaning that it helps build) hormone and increases the anabolic response to exercise

PROGESTERONE: YOUR CALMING FRIEND

Progesterone is primarily released from the ovaries during the second part of your menstrual cycle and is necessary in preparing your body for pregnancy. In fact, the literal translation of "progesterone" is "promoting gestation." If you become pregnant, progesterone helps nourish your uterus to carry the embryo through pregnancy. The body decides it's not much use to you in menopause, though, so since it's time to stop procreating, progesterone is no longer needed.

Progesterone also promotes a calming effect, reducing anxiety, mood swings, and irritability. It can also promote sleep, so declining levels of progesterone are typically accompanied by insomnia, a lower tolerance for stress, and increased anxiety. Although progesterone is mainly produced in the ovaries, some progesterone is produced in the brain.

Before menopause, the body will buffer the stress hormone cortisol with progesterone. Once those levels of progesterone go down, that buffering effect also declines, making it more difficult to cope with stress. Yeah, no shit, Sherlock!

Roles of progesterone in your body:

- Helps to prepare your body for conception and pregnancy

- Is a critical part of the menstrual cycle, promoting regular ovulation and increasing the chances of becoming pregnant

- Plays a part in sexual desire

- Promotes the growth of milk-producing glands in the breasts during pregnancy in preparation for breastfeeding

- Is necessary for the successful implantation of the fertilized egg in the uterus

- Offers benefits to breast health, cardiovascular health, bone health, and nervous system health, and most importantly brain function

TESTOSTERONE: YOUR SEX BUDDY

Testosterone is not just a male hormone. Yes, ladies, you have testosterone too, just in lower amounts than men. It is produced by both the ovaries and adrenal glands. It makes us a little horny, giving us that feeling of well-being, as well as increased energy, and helps us stay strong. Chances are if you build lean muscle easily, you have a healthy volume of testosterone.

As levels of estrogen and progesterone decline, you may reach a stage during your menopause transition when you have more testosterone relative to estrogen and progesterone. That's when you may see a shift in your distribution of body fat from a pear shape to a more predominantly apple shape as you gain belly fat.

Roles of testosterone in your body:

- Works with estrogen and progesterone to keep bones strong and healthy

- Keeps us feeling horny, and drives our desire and energy for sex

- Helps promote cognitive health

Too much of this hormone, known as free testosterone, along with increased estrogen can lead to polycystic ovarian syndrome (PCOS), a condition that interferes with monthly periods and the body's ability to ovulate, and which may make it harder for women to become pregnant.

My preference is to keep the information on these hormones very basic: one, because I am not a doctor, and two, because I think it's more important to understand that our declining sex hormones, the food we eat, the actions we take, and the exercise we perform all affect one another. While much of our hormonal health is out of our control, not all of it is! You can control things like cortisol (your stress hormone) and insulin (your fat, sugar, and vitamin-storage hormone); we'll cover this later in the book.

AHOY THERE, SYMPTOMS!

No one woman will experience this time of life exactly the same way as another. In this way it's a unique journey, but it's also a shared journey in its essence, meaning that it can be eased by knowing you are not going through this alone.

Menopause comes with a lot of potential symptoms—the list below is just a start. When these symptoms hit you like a thunderbolt, it feels like you're entering the menopocalypse. Nobody but you can truly appreciate what it feels like in your body. Sure, you'll get the nodding heads from your fellow menopausing witches—we are, after all, in this coven together. Yet you alone get to experience your very own menopocalypse hell. You feel like you can't remember a time when you felt well, and then when the symptoms subside slightly, you can't remember how awful they were. Still, the power of sharing your symptoms with others can help you immensely; realizing you are not alone in your suffering can ease the burden tremendously.

As a fit and healthy woman in her forties, I was surprised to struggle with most of the symptoms listed below. But menopause does not discriminate; as with many other health issues, much of it is out of our control. Genetics plays a major role in determining the age you enter perimenopause. NAMS confirms there is an association between the age you enter perimenopause and the age your mother did.

But genetics doesn't tell the whole story. Although I entered menopause around the same age as my mother did, my own menopause experience has been nothing like hers; she had only a few symptoms and seemed to sail on through. Many women assume they'll have a similar experience to that of their mothers, but that may not necessarily be the case. Factors that may contribute to your symptoms are the environment (say, if you live at a high altitude), lifestyle (for example, being a heavy smoker), or pure shitty bad luck (that's me!). Scientists are still looking at the genetic markers related to symptoms, and the answers are probably still a long way off.

I am still confused about why I struggled so much. I often think that if I had entered perimenopause overweight, with poor health markers, I would've been in a much worse state, as women with these characteristics statistically do struggle with more symptoms. It seems I'm just one of the lucky 25 percent of women who have extreme symptoms during the menopause journey that severely affect our quality of life, and we might never know why.

Common symptoms that women struggle with include:

- Irregular periods

- Stress and/or urge incontinence

- Depression

- Vaginal dryness

- Hot flashes

- Sleep problems (from insomnia to utter fatigue)

- Mood changes (like batshit crazy mood changes)

- Weight gain and slowed metabolism, with a slow but steady growth of a flesh blanket over your tummy

- Loss of breast fullness or the opposite—a growth of the largest pair of boobs you've ever owned

- Short-term memory loss and other cognitive impairments

- Night sweats

- Migraines and severe headaches

- Fatigue

- Anxiety

- Loss of sex drive or the opposite (on very rare occasions), where you're desperate to have sex with somebody, anybody!

- Bloating and flatulence, food sensitivities, and all that shit

- Psychological changes such as loss of self-confidence, feelings of invisibility, and isolation

Some lesser-known symptoms that are also associated with menopause are:

- Hearing problems/tinnitus

- Worsening allergies

- Tingling extremities/pins and needles

- Palpitations

- Burning tongue

- Bleeding gums

- Breast pain

- Formication (I said "formication," not "fornication"!); this is a sensation like ants crawling over your skin

- Hair loss (except for the white fuzz on your face)

- Cold flashes—the evil sister to hot flashes

- Loss of mojo and general zest for life

As you can see, the list just keeps on going, and I am pretty sure this isn't an exhaustive one. I compiled this from my own experience, medical texts, and experiences that other women have shared with me.

Not every symptom has a remedy. These symptoms are part of a process that your body has to go through, so part of the journey is learning to live with the new you and all of its baggage. There are many ways you can lessen the burden or even wipe out some of the worst symptoms, but we're not trying to fix anything here. The goal is to live your best menopause life! There are no quick-fix solutions, but there are real ways to feel better, stronger, and happier.

Menopause is so individual that it is almost impossible to tell how it will feel for you. As a result, there isn't a one-size-fits-all approach to this unique experience. I have talked to thousands of women, and although we can all empathize with and relate to one another, chances are we are not experiencing exactly the same thing, and therefore the same approaches may not work for all of us.

That is precisely what makes menopause so bloody frustrating. You might be having a symptom that isn't listed above, and then you are left asking: Is this menopause or just midlife? The best way to understand the journey of menopause is to talk to other women in your family or your community and ask them what they're experiencing or have experienced.

In a recent poll I created within my own online menopause community on Facebook, *Menopausing So Hard*, we came up with the top eight symptoms the women in that group experienced. Here they are, in no particular order:

FATIGUE

I remember feeling so tired I wanted to cry. And it wasn't because I wasn't getting a good night's sleep. I was clocking nine to ten hours each night on average. Yet each day I just wanted to crash out cold. It made absolutely no sense to me when I was nailing my workouts and my nutrition was on point, as were my recovery and stress levels.

So why did I feel this utter fatigue? Our fluctuating hormones cause insomnia, in addition to hot flashes, mood swings, and cognitive functioning issues. These fluctuating hormones can also totally disrupt our energy levels.

This type of debilitating fatigue doesn't seem to be eased by resting or napping and can be made much worse by exercise and too much mental stimulation. If you add in other symptoms like insomnia and hot flashes, or other conditions you may have such as depression and anxiety, you have a big bag of fucked-up-ness. Fatigue levels can also be increased by smoking, drinking, being sedentary (yes, I know I am contradicting myself; I said exercise can make fatigue worse and now I am saying *not* exercising does the same. Welcome to menopause!), and overindulging in junk food.

Chronic fatigue syndrome (CFS) is an extreme example of such fatigue; it's a medically recognized condition but is not easily identifiable. A study by the U.S. Centers for Disease Control and Prevention showed a link between CFS and early menopause. A sample of eighty-four women with CFS was compared with a control group of seventy-three healthy women. Although this strikes me as a particularly small number to use as a basis for making sweeping statements, the study did show that women in their forties and fifties—which is when women are experiencing menopause—are four times as likely to suffer from CFS as women in other age groups.

We also know that missing our happy hormonal friend estrogen can contribute to fatigue. Reduced levels of estrogen mean a surge in cortisol, which is known to bring on fatigue.

COGNITIVE DIFFICULTIES

Another major problem for me and others in my community was short-term memory loss. Menopause zombie brain sucks big time. I would sometimes forget the most basic words, mid-sentence, and then would be unable to finish because I'd have forgotten what I was talking about. It is so frustrating to live like that, and it's humiliating to feel stupid or scatterbrained in front of others, especially when you already feel invisible. In addition, organization, planning, and concentration can become troublesome, even if you have previously excelled at these things.

The sudden inability to remember the most basic things is so scary that women often panic that they might have Alzheimer's. Lisa Mosconi, a neuroscientist at Weill Cornell Medical College, is researching the link between menopause and Alzheimer's, which affects twice as many women as men. In a recent interview with the website Medium, Mosconi said, "Estrogen is a strong neuroprotective hormone. It's strongly associated with the immune system, it's a neuroplastic hormone, so if you lose it, your brain starts aging faster." The research continues, but Mosconi emphasizes the importance of exercise, nutrition, and stress management to help counter some of the symptoms of menopause zombie brain.

A few years ago, when my older son and I were watching my younger son play in a basketball game, my older son reminded me of when he also played middle-school basketball. For the life of me I couldn't remember that at all, and he spent thirty minutes trying to refresh my memory, to no avail. Finally, he conceded that either I was a terrible parent for not remembering or I had dementia. Either way he was worried. It completely felt like a senior moment. Eventually, after I looked at some old photos, it all came back to me. But the whole situation unnerved me.

A study of dementia undertaken by the University of Colorado School of Medicine concluded that the cognitive symptoms that feel extreme in menopausal women seem to peak in the late stages of perimenopause, and that they are separate from natural aging. During postmenopause, memory improves. I am now writing a book, but just four years ago I could barely write my shopping list—and then if I did manage to do so, I'd forget where I put it.

Eating well, moving often, and managing stress, along with HT if you're a candidate, can help with these neurological symptoms. Part 2 of this book is dedicated to showing you how to do this. Always stay focused on your health, and should you be overly concerned about something, then go and see your doctor. Have faith that this too shall pass.

DEPRESSION

I can speak about depression from experience. Although I have a pretty good outlook on life, I have also experienced some pretty rough personal stuff over the years that could have sent anybody into a downward spiral, and I always prided myself on being one of those people who could stay positive even when everything was going haywire.

I was already fed up with feeling unwell in general as a result of perimenopause, but after a while I started to feel numb, bored, lifeless, and utterly fatigued. Initially, I thought it was my marriage. I thought I was bored with my husband, maybe bored with the kids, and, quite frankly, bored with myself. It really took a long time for me to sit back and see that I wouldn't change any part of my life if I could, so there must have been another reason I was feeling that way.

Everybody noticed, including my kids. They were worried about me. I wasn't myself and I wasn't reaching my potential by any stretch. I had always been that person who kept busy with a laundry list of projects and errands, and thrived on it. Now I could barely do one thing each day; it was soul-destroying. I wasn't present. Everybody around me was affected.

When my gynecologist diagnosed depression caused by severely low estrogen, I literally jumped up in the air and kissed him. I had an answer. I wasn't going crazy. I'd known there had to be a reason I was feeling that way, and now I knew what it was. I had a chemical imbalance that was out of my control, and the resulting depression wasn't something I could simply talk my way out of—it was much bigger than that. My body was not coping with the changes that were happening.

The worst thing about being diagnosed with depression, though, was the fact that I didn't want to be diagnosed with depression! I felt almost ashamed and embarrassed by it. I opted to take a specific antidepressant that is often prescribed for menopause, and it kept my depression at bay. But it also protected my silence; I thought that if I told people about my struggles, they would see them as a sign of failing. Taking an antidepressant helped me get a handle on the depression, and I was able to keep that secret to myself.

My life turned around the minute I started taking the pills, and as an off-label benefit, they also managed both my migraines and hot flashes. After two years, I no longer needed to take the pills, but they got me through one of the hardest periods of my life.

I had to work hard to eliminate the stigma and shame that I associated with depression and taking antidepressants. I didn't want my kids to see my negative attitude toward mental health issues. That's why I now choose to speak openly about my struggles, a choice that has helped the connection in my family grow stronger.

There are many options for treating depression, and you have to decide what route you want to take. Women are routinely prescribed antidepressants during this time. Hormone therapy should actually be considered the first line of treatment, but lack of knowledge and awareness about mental health struggles during perimenopause prevents this from happening. In addition to pharmaceutical solutions, lifestyle factors like exercise, diet, stress management, and mindset can and should play a huge role in your treatment. These lifestyle factors are the keystones of my work and are discussed in Part 2 of this book.

ANXIETY

An example of the extreme anxiety I experienced during perimenopause occurred during a vacation I had planned with my family at an all-inclusive resort in the Dominican Republic. Sounds awesome right? Only it wasn't. It was a bad choice for this family, who much prefer to get out and explore than to lie on a beach. Regardless, one of my strengths is the ability to make the best of it.

Only this time it all went wrong. On day one I experienced a panic attack, for the second time in my life. It started with my feeling trapped in resort jail. Soon my heart was racing, I couldn't catch my breath, and I was on the verge of breaking down.

I knew that increased anxiety was a common symptom of menopause, but I wasn't in control of what was happening to me.

Deep breathing, crying, sleeping, and walking didn't help me. So I went to the hotel gym and started running on the treadmill. A slow, plodding six miles later, the anxiety lifted. I understand now what people mean when they tell me that they feel like they're dying or having a heart attack when a panic attack strikes—it is no joke.

This was my perimenopause.

When panic or anxiety strike, it's up to you to find what works best for you. Running calms me down, but something else might work for you.

The definition of anxiety is a feeling of worry, nervousness, or unease, typically about an imminent event or something with an uncertain outcome. This description intimates that your symptoms are all psychological, that you might resolve them by focusing on your mental well-being. What royally pisses me off is the lack of discussion of the crippling physical manifestations of anxiety.

On another occasion, when I was writing an article for my blog, I had an anxiety attack and proceeded to describe it as I continued writing: "I'm currently typing this article with a crushing feeling in my chest that won't abate. I'm struggling to catch my breath and hate myself for not being able to make this subside, no matter how many belly breaths I do. It's making my temples throb and my neck is stiff, it's so tiring. The pain is visceral; it extends past my chest down my arms and leaves me with trembling hands like I've drunk too much coffee."

As your hormones fluctuate in perimenopause, there will be times when estrogen is high, and this can make cortisol levels rise. You need to make friends with both depression and anxiety—after all, you are in this together. Depression is often associated with living in the past, focusing on how things might have been. Anxiety is often associated with worrying about the future and having no control over what might happen. It's easy to get so hung up on a future event that you miss what's right in front of you, in the here and now. Learning to be present, to be mindful and live fully in the moment, is a game-changer for managing both depression and anxiety. Chapter 9 discusses this in more detail.

Speaking with a therapist can be a great help in putting things in perspective. Don't assume that because your hormones are out partying that working on your body-mind connection is a lost cause.

If you are a lifelong sufferer of either depression or anxiety, some of your symptoms may be heightened during menopause. It's worth being aware of this so that when you speak to your doctor you can come up with a strategy to deal with it, whether through additional medication or through counseling. Other strategies that can be part of your healing are mindfulness, meditation, exercise, diet, and stress management—all covered in Part 2 of this book.

WEIGHT GAIN

Oh dear—the flesh blanket that is marshmallow menopause tummy. Except for when I was pregnant, I have weighed exactly the same since the age of sixteen. So when I came back from my summer holidays ten pounds heavier than ever, I was gutted. My body had stopped forgiving me for my indulgences!

I have always been a pretty healthy eater who still enjoys her treats, and I love looking after the health of my body, so why—after all the time, effort, and goodness that I had given my body—did it feel like it was betraying me?

Changes in estrogen levels affect the distribution of fat deposits in the body, moving fat more predominantly to the belly area. Now let me clarify: hormonal changes didn't make me extra curvy—it's the cream cakes and bacon sandwiches that did that. But the way my body reacted to these indulgences had definitely changed. Whereas in the past I could get away with occasional treats, now my body just said no! I had to start being more strategic and mindful about my eating.

Menopause not only changes the shape of your body but also causes increased water and gas retention. Sometimes the fullness or tightness you feel from these symptoms can make you feel heavier and larger than you are. This is probably one of the most upsetting things for women to cope with. It can really knock your self-confidence to have extra weight hanging around your belly, especially when despite all your best efforts, nothing seems to get rid of it. But as frustrating as the flesh blanket is, there are ways to get it under control, again discussed in Part 2.

As mentioned earlier in this chapter, about 20 percent of women will gain at least ten pounds throughout their menopause journey, but that doesn't make losing weight impossible. Weight loss in menopause is a multifaceted problem that requires an in-depth discussion. Head over to Chapter 5, where I spill the beans about why we gain weight and what we can do about it.

INCONTINENCE

One day on a five-kilometer run in the hilly beauty of Scotland, I looked down at my leggings and saw that they were drenched. Yes, I had peed myself.

I was horrified. This had never happened to me before—and how could it? I'm a fitness trainer, and I had borne two kids years before and had never experienced anything like this. Skipping, trampolining, jumping, sneezing, and coughing had never been an issue for me in the years following my two births, yet at the age of forty-four I was peeing myself on a run. I was devastated, as well as embarrassed.

I immediately went to see a pelvic-health physiotherapist for help. I knew this condition was common. But I also knew that it wasn't normal and that I didn't need to accept it.

My pelvic-health physiotherapist gave me an internal examination, which provided tactile feedback that really helped me understand what was happening. Pelvic-floor health is a big topic, but very often it's not discussed at all. I mean, who wants to talk about peeing their pants? Yet the numbers show that more than 46 percent of women experience incontinence, and that's only those who report it.

After some therapy, which included manual manipulation and at-home exercises, my condition improved significantly. Interestingly enough, my pelvic-health physio never suggested a connection between my incontinence and perimenopause.

Reduced estrogen can to lead to reduced collagen in your connective tissue, which means these tissues aren't as elastic as they once were (hence the wrinkles on your face). It can also affect the strength and function of the pelvic floor as a whole, making you struggle with vaginal dryness, incontinence, and painful sex. This condition is commonly known as vaginal atrophy, but because the condition causes both vaginal and urinary symptoms, medical professionals use the term "genitourinary syndrome of menopause" (GSM). This is a unique area of physiotherapy and many women need to learn or relearn how to correctly strengthen their pelvic floor. This topic is more fully discussed in Chapter 4.

MIGRAINES AND SEVERE HEADACHES

The worst of my symptoms was migraines. Now that I have a label for what I was struggling with, I have learned how to manage them. It took a lot of experimenting with foods, medication, and relaxation methods to reduce stress, which is a huge contributor to migraines. I encourage you to become a detective for your own health so that you can find the right course of treatment for you. I still occasionally suffer from migraines, but they are less intense. There's also some relief in knowing that in general migraine intensity lessens as we reach the postmenopause stage.

Migraines suck! They have left me and millions of women incapacitated because of their severity. Of the 28 million Americans who suffer from migraines, 70 percent of them are women. There is a definite estrogen connection, but scientists are still trying to work out why they occur. And because we all experience menopause differently, the severity or occurrence of related migraines can't be accurately determined.

Women who suffer from migraines see a drop in their quality of life. Migraines can affect both their work and their home life and can lead to depression. Migraines are often undiagnosed (again I put my hand up here) and inappropriately treated; in fact, many of the symptoms of migraine don't feel like a migraine. I suffered from migraine with aura but never got a headache. Instead I was overcome with vertigo, nausea, vision and hearing problems, and some cognitive confusion.

The statistics are on our side though, ladies; most studies show that after we reach menopause and head on into postmenopause, the symptoms subside and may even vanish—hooray!

Stress, lack of sleep, hormonal fluctuations, some foods, and alcohol are known triggers of migraines, so it's worth you spending the time to identify your triggers. I had to stop drinking, which was a bummer for me, and to limit the coffee I drank. In addition, there is pharmaceutical treatment available for migraines, which includes HT. As always, it's best to speak to your medical professional about what is best for you.

HOT FLASHES/NIGHT SWEATS/COLD FLASHES

Hot flashes, night sweats, and cold flashes all are classified as vasomotor symptoms. "Vasomotor" refers to the changing temperature of the body. These are the symptoms that are most often associated with menopause, yet we know very little about why women struggle with them during menopause. Current theories point to changes in your estrogen levels, which appear to affect your hypothalamus, the part of your brain that is responsible for regulating your body's temperature. Anywhere from 75 to 85 percent of women in North America will struggle with hot flashes, which are often accompanied by excessive sweating and increased heart rate.

At the 2019 North American Menopause Society conference, psychiatry professor Rebecca Thurston presented her research showing the link between frequent hot flashes and an increased risk of cardiovascular disease. "What we found," she said, "is that women with more frequent hot flashes when they entered into the study in their mid-forties had double the risk of heart attacks, strokes, and heart failure later in life." So hot flashes are clearly not just an inconvenient symptom of menopause; they may also affect your overall health.

The good news is there are a few treatments and strategies you can take to help reduce the severity of hot flashes. Medical organizations and experts agree that HT is the best treatment available for reducing the severity of symptoms. Nonpharmaceutical options include evening primrose oil and black cohosh supplements, but the data is currently mixed on their effectiveness. Some foods can trigger hot flashes, as can alcohol, stress, and lack of sleep. Again, this is an opportunity for you to take control of your lifestyle to help alleviate the severity of your symptoms.

I'M SURE YOU'RE thinking, bloody hell, I had no idea symptoms could be so varied and severe. Many women feel this way. I recently did an interview with *Woman's Day* in which I spoke openly about my menopausal depression.

Within a week I had over three thousand women contact me to say they or their doctor had never associated depression with menopause. When you can finally identify your symptoms and put a name to them, then you can start to take action. The worst thing in the world is to feel unwell or symptomatic without having any answers. This is your chance to be your own menopause advocate, and I will help you along the way.

— 2 —

THE GOOD, THE BAD, AND THE UGLY OF HT (PLUS OTHER TREATMENT OPTIONS)

I T WOULD BE impossible to write a book about menopause without mentioning hormone therapy (HT). HT has had a bad rap for a long time. Women are often petrified of it because of the associated risk of breast cancer and other diseases. And if they do decide to take it, they have to decide whether they should take bioidentical or traditional HT. And should they use gels, patches, pellets, or cream? Or should they skip it altogether and rely on acupuncture or black cohosh, which is a heavily marketed over-the-counter remedy? Seriously, it is a bloody minefield out there; I don't blame women for being utterly confused.

In addition, some women feel ashamed of looking for treatment for what is just another "natural process." Seventy-five percent of women will have menopause symptoms.

At least 15 to 20 percent of women experience extreme symptoms that alter their quality of life but they never consider HT, yet the evidence shows that it's often a life-transforming treatment. I often hear women say things like, "I'm resisting taking hormones," or "I've finally given in and decided to try them." This type of narrative is very harmful. Shrouding HT in a shameful cloak is not doing any women a favor, and we must stop talking this way.

In medical terms, hormone replacement therapy (HRT) is the treatment offered to women who enter menopause *before* the age of forty; the treatment is typically a fairly high dose of estrogen and progesterone, sometimes in the form of a birth control pill. Hormone therapy (without the "R") is given to women over the age of forty whose bloodwork suggests declining hormones, or over the age of forty-five if they have presenting symptoms, and is typically a lower dose of both estrogen and progesterone. Most women use the acronym HRT when referring to their treatment, but the more correct and currently accepted name is HT. The terminology HT moves away from the idea that we are replacing hormones and implies that the treatment is instead a method of supporting hormones, thus removing that element of shame.

HT is used not only for the treatment of menopausal symptoms but also as a long-term way to prevent diseases that occur as a result of declining estrogen. Some menopause specialists recommend it as treatment for conditions such as brain fog, mood disorders, thinning hair, and metabolic syndrome, although this practice is still somewhat controversial even among experts.

HT can reduce the risk of cardiovascular disease, especially if you start HT within ten years of menopause. It can also help lower cholesterol levels. Heart disease is currently the leading cause of death in women, affecting one in five women. HT can also prevent and reverse bone loss as a result of osteopenia and possibly of osteoporosis.

Other studies indicate that HT can help reduce type 2 diabetes, some cancers, and possibly Alzheimer's, a disease that many women fear the most. At the Alzheimer's Association International Conference in early 2020, two studies were presented that showed a correlation between female hormones and the disease. The studies found that HT may help if women get it at the right time; more research is currently under way.

So why is there so much reluctance to even consider HT as a viable treatment?

THE CONTROVERSY OVER HT

In 2002, the Women's Health Institute (WHI) published a study looking into the benefits of taking HT to prevent heart disease if given as primary prevention. The study was not designed to look at estrogen as a treatment for symptomatic hot flashes. This study was considered the gold standard of all studies looking into the benefits of taking HT to prevent heart disease.

Women were randomly given hormones or a placebo for what was to be a fifteen-year period, but the study was stopped early when the researchers saw an increase in a number of diseases, including breast cancer, heart disease, and stroke. The conclusion was that HT should not be prescribed; the risks were too grave. When my own mother went through menopause, the WHI report had just been released, and I told her that under no circumstances was she to take hormones, believing that hormones did increase the risk of breast cancer. Following the release of the study, U.S. sales of Premarin, an estrogen-based hormone derived from pregnant mares' urine, dropped from $2 billion to $880 million.

In their groundbreaking 2018 book *Estrogen Matters*, Avrum Bluming, MD, and Carol Tavris, PhD, share their exhaustive research into the original WHI study. They found many errors in its conclusions that HT is harmful. They explain that as a result of the study, the new mantra has been that if women are going to take postmenopausal estrogen (since it *does* help so many), they should take "the smallest dose for the shortest time." They give evidence that there is no scientific basis to this recommendation. Rather, they say that it was merely an "uncomfortable compromise" from physicians who knew HT helped many women.

NAMS has backed this up with the following position statement: "The concept of 'lowest dose for the shortest period of time' may be inadequate or even harmful for some women. A more fitting concept is 'appropriate dose, duration, regimen, and route of administration.'"

Over time, the study has been re-examined and post-hoc analysis has been published using the original data. It turns out that the WHI rushed the report to publication before the researchers of the study even had time to read the draft; one of the researchers has since published a blistering account of how the study violated the scientific process. The upshot of this has been an agreement that taking HT does *not* significantly increase the risk of breast cancer; the risk was not statistically significant compared with known lifestyle risk factors such as smoking, obesity, and being overweight.

So why hasn't estrogen been fully vindicated? Why do women still believe that HT causes breast cancer?

It's fair to say that we tend to hang onto scary shit, even if it quite possibly is misinformation. At an evolutionary level, fear is a great motivator. For example, if we fear we might be at (real or perceived) risk of a disease, we will find ways to overcome those risks by taking decisive healthy actions. Our actions might be worthless, but the fear in us drives us to try to somehow take control.

In her book *Perimenopower*, Katarina Wilk talks about the tendency for us to cling to the risks. Cognitive psychologist Daniel Kahneman calls this "theory-induced blindness," in which adherence to a theory makes people unable to see its flaws or accept new evidence. I know in the past I have been wary of changing my mind because I didn't want to be seen as inconsistent or incorrect. But that way of thinking is flawed if we are to continue to expand our knowledge. There have been times when I have just had to swallow my pride and admit that I was wrong. (Never to my husband though. Remember: we are never wrong when it comes to that fight!)

CLEARING UP MISCONCEPTIONS

Dr. Louise Newson, a menopause expert from the U.K., is doing an amazing job of clearing up some of the misconceptions about HT and finding the right treatment for women. "So many women I see in my clinic are worried about taking HT because of their perceived breast cancer

risk," she told me. "Yet experiencing menopausal symptoms (such as low mood, reduced energy, joint pains, and
poor sleep) has led them to increase their weight, drink
more alcohol, do less exercise. All these lifestyle factors
increase their future risk of breast cancer usually without
them realizing it; yet taking HT is associated with a lower
risk of breast cancer than these lifestyle changes. Women
often thank me, as taking HT gives them their lives back;
they usually have more energy and are happier. This usually means that their lifestyle improves so they exercise
more, eat a more healthy diet, and drink less alcohol. So
even with taking HT, they have a lower future risk of breast
cancer than they had before."

There are many different types of HT, and you should
work with your doctor to find which will work best for
you. As with any medication you take, there will be risks,
and therefore you must discuss them. The risks that most
commonly freak out women are breast cancer, stroke, and
blood clots. These risks, however, have been deemed to
be small compared with the benefits. Let's put this into
perspective: the risk of breast cancer using HT is similar
to the risk of breast cancer for women who are obese or
drink alcohol daily.

So does that mean that HT is right for you?

It depends. Crappy response, I know, but this is a decision that you and your doctor must make together based
on a number of factors, including your age, health status,
and genetics, the type of HT to be taken, and the length
of use. For example, if you're a breast cancer survivor you
may be sensitive to estrogen in your system, so the current
recommendation from NAMS is that nonhormonal therapies should be your first approach. Yet some breast cancers

respond positively to estrogen, in which case you might be a candidate for HT. The decision needs to be individualized and all risks and benefits taken into account, including quality of life, not just the risk that breast cancer will recur, which might be very low. This is why it is important to have full, frank discussions with your primary health care provider.

The current guidelines tell us that the window of opportunity for HT is when you're under the age of sixty, within ten years since your last period. This is when you will get most benefits from the treatment, and from that point you can stay on the treatment for as long as you want to. Some women never come off HT because of the health benefits (there are women in their seventies and eighties who take it), and some women come off HT once their symptoms seem to have subsided; that decision is something to discuss with your doctor. If you are over sixty or more than ten years past your last period, it may still be an option, but your doctor will need to do a risk assessment to see if you're a candidate.

If you are struggling to find adequate treatment from your doctor, it may be because they haven't had specific training in menopause. In fact, most doctors don't have any; only 20 percent of ob-gyn residency programs provide any menopause training at all. It's simply shocking that you might seek out a gynecologist who ends up having no knowledge of menopause. This only reinforces the message that we are the forgotten patients. NAMS is trying to right this wrong, and it maintains a list of certified menopause specialists on its website (menopause.org). Hopefully there's one in your area.

"Nearly one-third of this country's women are post-menopausal," says gynecologist Wen Shen, an assistant professor in the Johns Hopkins Department of Gynecology and Obstetrics. "Many of them are needlessly suffering."

You do not need to suffer.

For many of the women I interviewed for this book, HT has completely changed their lives. It has helped to manage most of their symptoms and given them renewed vigor and energy. I have already told you about the wondrous things estrogen can do, and reintroducing it into your menopausing life might be what prevents you from going bonkers.

I think HT saved me. I wish I had started sooner. [I'm] thankful for my doctor, who encouraged me to be open-minded. My tiny little dose has literally turned my life around. I literally felt and saw the evidence of how important hormones are to how we function and feel.

TAMMY PENNINGTON,
Menopausing So Hard member

HT usually involves a combination of both estrogen and progesterone. Doctors will not prescribe estrogen alone if you still have your uterus, as estrogen will thicken the lining of the uterus, causing a higher risk of uterine cancer. In that case HT will always be prescribed with a progesterone, which reverses this risk. If you no longer have a uterus, you can be prescribed estrogen only. Hormones come in a number of preparations. Estrogen is typically a gel, a patch, or an oral medication. It can also come in a cream or tablet for localized use in the vagina to treat vaginal atrophy (which is discussed in Chapter 4). Progesterone is added either by tablet or through an intrauterine device (IUD); its purpose again is to protect your uterus. There are also preparations that combine both, available in both patch and tablet. There has been shown to be a slight increased risk—and I mean minutely small—of clots when taking oral estrogen; some doctors prefer to offer the transdermal (i.e., delivered through the skin) alternatives of patch or gel. But one size does not fit all, and this should not change your decision unless you are truly at increased risk of blood clots. In fact, if you ever took birth control tablets or were pregnant you assumed a much higher risk of blood clots than you do with the use of hormone therapy.

"BIOIDENTICAL" HORMONES ARE NOT ALWAYS REGULATED

Many of us prefer to interfere with nature as little as possible and would rather take a safe and effective plant-based remedy instead of a chemically produced substance. The marketers of unregulated bioidentical hormones know this—and are using this fact as a marketing strategy, misleading women globally. "Bioidentical" simply means manufactured hormones similar in structure to the hormones your body produces. The term was created by compounding pharmacies to promote the unregulated hormones they produce.

The term has been widely adopted now, as in the U.S. we see both FDA-regulated and nonregulated (i.e., produced by a compounding pharmacy) bioidentical hormones. In the U.K., the terms have become so muddled that regulated bioidentical hormones, which must be prescribed by a doctor, now use the term *body-identical* instead.

Add to this the fact that you can buy hormones on Amazon, just as you might buy shampoo. The whole situation is confusing, isn't it? Let's examine the claims made by marketers of unregulated bioidentical hormones.

Claim: The marketers of unregulated bioidentical hormones claim that their hormones are safer than FDA-approved drugs.

Evidence: The FDA website says, "Compounded drugs are not FDA-approved. This means that FDA does not verify the safety or effectiveness of compounded drugs. Consumers and health professionals rely on the drug approval process for verification of safety, effectiveness, and quality. Compounded drugs also lack an FDA finding of manufacturing quality before such drugs are marketed." This is a position supported by the Endocrine Society, NAMS, and most other medical bodies.

The claims for compounded bioidentical hormones are simply not supported by the evidence. Across the Atlantic, the British Menopause Society (BMS) says that the term "bioidentical hormones" is misleading and that women should take only regulated HT, which includes hormones that are natural and identical to those produced in your body.

Claim: Unregulated bioidentical hormones are completely natural.

Evidence: Unregulated bioidenticals are about as natural as Dolly Parton's tits. One of the selling points of these hormones is that they're derived from yams or soy and are therefore said to be natural. But they're still chemically produced; they're still made in a lab. In fact, FDA-approved bioidentical HT is *also* derived from plants and so could also be considered "natural" by that definition. The difference is that the latter is regulated and approved by governing bodies.

Claim: Compounding pharmacy bioidenticals are as effective as regulated hormones.

Evidence: Bioidentical hormones are made by a compounding pharmacist and are not approved by the FDA. As already mentioned, it is possible to buy these products online or over the counter, rather than through a prescription from your doctor. The quality and quantity of the hormones you are taking are then at the whim of the manufacturer. As a result, you don't know what the side effects might be or how effective the hormones will be. These hormones also tend to be more costly. I know women who have spent thousands of dollars on unregulated hormones when there were readily available regulated alternatives at a fraction of the price.

The latest trend in private clinics seems to be to encourage women to have "bioidentical hormone pellets" implanted in their skin. These pellets are expensive, lack regulated testing, and have been associated with adverse effects, which include endometrial cancer, strokes, heart attacks, deep vein thrombosis, cellulitis, and pellet extrusion. The company that produces these pellets is currently under investigation by the FDA. Why would you choose to take hormones that could be a risk to your health when there are safer and cheaper options available from your doctor?

Claim: Unregulated bioidentical hormones are not drugs because they have the same molecular structure as hormones found naturally in the body.

Evidence: Unregulated bioidentical hormones are most definitely drugs. They are made in a lab and mixed together by a pharmacist. And while they may have the same molecular structure as your body's hormones, so does FDA-approved bioidentical HT, and only the latter will be tested for efficacy and safety.

Claim: Unregulated bioidentical hormones have no long-term health risks.

Evidence: There is simply no reliable evidence to back up this claim as no long-term studies have been undertaken; we don't know their long-term impacts. There is simply not enough scrutiny, as there is with regulated HT, which is currently the best-documented and most effective treatment for menopause.

A STATEMENT FROM the American College of Obstetricians and Gynecologists (ACOG) concludes: "Customized compounded hormones pose additional risks. These preparations have variable purity and potency and lack efficacy and safety data. Because of variable bioavailability and bioactivity, both underdosage and overdosage are possible."

Take my advice: save your money by not buying these expensive, inconsistent options. Personally, I think it's simple; don't use hormones from an unregulated source and don't buy hormones online. Use regulated hormones only, and make sure you get them from your doctor.

OTHER PHARMACEUTICAL TREATMENT OPTIONS

ANTIDEPRESSANTS

HT should be offered as the first option to manage your symptoms. Many doctors, however (who are likely not educated about menopause), prescribe antidepressants as an initial treatment. Some antidepressants do in fact offer some off-label benefits—for example, relief from vasomotor symptoms such as hot flashes and night sweats—and they can be a valid option for some women who are not candidates for HT.

The problem is when women who are valid candidates for HT are offered antidepressants instead. I initially opted to take an antidepressant called Venlafaxine instead of HT, which really helped with my mental health symptoms, but it didn't help with *all* my symptoms. For example, I still struggled with incontinence, fatigue, and my tanked libido. The only thing that really worked for me was HT.

I should add that there are some women who take both HT and antidepressants, and there may be underlying mental health issues that HT alone cannot resolve. You should talk to your doctor to find the nuanced treatment that works best for you.

TESTOSTERONE

Some doctors may also offer you testosterone in addition to your HT. Testosterone is produced in both the ovaries and the adrenal glands, and if your levels dip too low, you may benefit from a supplemental dose. This is usually established by a blood test ordered by your doctor. Low testosterone can cause fatigue, lack of sex drive, and impaired cognitive ability that aren't resolved when you take estrogen and progesterone. Unfortunately, it's very easy to get testosterone from unregulated sources, so if you require it as part of your treatment plan, you should take the advice of your medical team. Most doctors agree that the main reason to take testosterone is low libido that is bothersome and causes distress to the woman.

ALTERNATIVE/COMPLEMENTARY REMEDIES

So far in this chapter, we've discussed what the science tells us about treatments that have been rigorously tested and subsequently regulated for safe use. In contrast, many alternative therapies are not regulated. Herbal supplements, for example, are often considered dietary supplements, which are classed as food rather than drugs. This means that manufacturers do not have to seek government approval before selling them.

Alternative herbs currently marketed for menopause symptoms include *adaptogens*, which are natural substances considered to help the body adapt to stress and to exert a normalizing effect on bodily processes. The most common adaptogens used for menopause are ashwagandha, maca, and schisandra. These are said to be helpful when you are struggling with cognitive issues, hot flashes, fatigue, or anxiety, and there is some research to corroborate these claims. Other marketed natural treatments for menopause are black cohosh and phytoestrogens derived from soy.

A word of caution: just because herbs are natural doesn't mean they're safe or effective. Some may interfere with other medications you're taking, they're usually expensive, and they don't always have quality studies to back up their claims. For example, black cohosh taken in excessive doses may cause liver toxicity, yet in Germany it is now a prescribed remedy for menopause, meaning that the claims about its effectiveness might be true but patients must speak with their doctors before taking it. I'm sure over time we will learn more about how these remedies work and what long-term impacts they can have on our bodies, but for now we don't have all of the information.

You also need to know that these supplements are not going to do the same job as HT. I see alternatives pushed on women as "positive" alternatives, which suggests that there's something negative about HT, which there is not. Many women in my community have tried these alternatives, some with success, but many report that they were expensive or that they were not always effective, especially if their menopausal symptoms were severe. Lastly, women who take these alternatives without medical supervision may be putting their health at risk.

It was only a matter of time before the tech companies would see an opportunity in the menopause crowd, and I don't think that's necessarily a bad thing. Menopausal women are a burden on the economy and the health care system, and tech-savvy Gen X women are looking for solutions that can help. Tech developments range from menopause tracking and meditation smartphone apps to online telemedicine services that let you speak directly to a trained menopause specialist, eliminating the need to go through any shenanigans with your doctor. There is also a commercially available product created by three MIT graduates who were working in over-air-conditioned spaces and wanted a way to regulate their own body temperature. It's a device you wear on your wrist, and you press a button to send hot or cold signals into your skin; research is currently being done to determine whether it can be helpful for women struggling with vasomotor symptoms.

KNOWING WHEN TO seek medical help during menopause can be difficult. Often the symptoms of menopause come and go, and by the time you go to the doctor you may feel okay. Sometimes trying to describe or even nail down how you're feeling and then relaying that information to a medical professional can be difficult. I have certainly felt that way.

Keeping a record of your symptoms can help.

MENOPAUSE TRACKER

Many women use apps to track their periods, so why not start tracking your menopause symptoms? There may be menopause apps on the market, but I'm old school and have found it helpful to simply write the data down. I found this strategy very useful when speaking to my gynecologist because it made sure I had that information on

hand. With your menopausing brain, you can have difficulty remembering what you felt like, so recording the
information is a useful tool. Being proactive is a great way
to take control of your health, and tracking your symptoms allows you to see where to focus.

I suggest tracking the following information.

- *Menstrual cycle:* date, length of cycle, flow (heavy or
  light), time between periods

- *Symptoms:* incontinence, insomnia, migraines, fatigue,
  painful sex, weight gain, joint pain, hot flashes, etc.

- *Emotional health:* anxiety, depression, panic attacks,
  mood swings

This is a great way for you to learn about your own body
and start to see patterns. Because my hormones were very
erratic and I wasn't having regular cycles, I couldn't associate my symptoms to "the time of the month," but I knew
that incontinence and migraines are associated with low
estrogen, so I could sort of track my cycle by those symptoms. Identifying this pattern helped me to control the
things that were within my control and to form a big picture to present to my doctor.

When talking to your doctor, don't hand him or her your
complete record. Rather, supply a summary of what you've
experienced over a three-to-six-month period. It might
look something like this:

DATE	MENSTRUAL CYCLE: Length of cycle, flow (heavy or light), time between periods	SYMPTOMS: Incontinence, insomnia, migraines, fatigue, painful sex, weight gain, joint pain, hot flashes, etc.	EMOTIONAL HEALTH: Anxiety, depression, panic attacks, mood swings	FOOD, MEDICINE, ACTIVITY: Dietary intolerance, GI issues, other medicines you take, your general activity level; record any info that might be helpful
Mar. 17	Started a 5-day cycle. Heavy with small clots.		Very low mood and fatigue	
Mar. 25	n/a	Migraine, fatigue, insomnia	Depressed	No appetite, took migraine medication at bedtime

MEETING WITH YOUR DOCTOR

The average time for a doctor's appointment in the U.S. and Canada is fifteen minutes, so you need to use it wisely. Armed with your concise list of symptoms obtained from your menopause tracker, you can make the most of your time. Here are some strategies to get ready for your appointment.

- Turn up on time and prepared for your appointment.

- Do your research (read this book!) before the appointment so that you have some knowledge about menopause.

- Decide in advance whether you're open to Western medicine, diet and lifestyle changes, supplements, or alternative therapies, and be open-minded when speaking to a medical professional.

- Remember, the symptoms you're experiencing may not be related to menopause. We can't blame it for everything!

Don't be afraid to advocate for your health. If you feel that your doctor cannot answer all your questions in one appointment, book a follow-up appointment. And if you don't get the answers you want, or you feel that your doctor is not the person to help you, ask for a referral to a medical professional who specializes in menopause.

QUESTIONS TO ASK YOUR DOCTOR

There are many ways to approach the conversation with your doctor, depending on your own specific needs. The doctor can tell you about options for treatment and blood tests, which will differ depending on your country, health care system, and finances (unfortunately). Again, don't be afraid to ask the questions and advocate for yourself. Consider asking:

- What treatments are available to you for perimenopause through postmenopause?

- What are the risks of taking the medication based on your personal history, genetics, and lifestyle?

- How long will you be on a suggested medication?

- When will you start to feel better?

- Should the doctor arrange a baseline hormonal test?

- Should you see a gynecologist for your treatment?

- Would a therapist help you with your depression, anxiety, mood swings?

- Would a pelvic-floor physiotherapist help you with incontinence?

As always, there are advantages and disadvantages to any treatment, whether it be HT or alternative medicine. We all have a unique chemical soup inside us that makes us react differently to treatments. As women advocating for our health, we must be informed and open-minded and be prepared to have a fulfilling and satisfying discussion with our doctors.

My personal experience was that HT was a necessity. I was initially reluctant to try it and instead took antidepressants for a few years, until they just didn't cut the mustard anymore. When I started peeing my pants and found my libido had got up and left me, I knew I needed to change my treatment. I also tried many different types of HT before I found the one that worked for me.

I don't believe HT to be a panacea; some women just do not do well on the treatment despite all their efforts. I had a very bad reaction to micronized progesterone, which is the oral medicine required to protect the uterus while taking estrogen therapy. It gave me severe feelings of depression and impending doom, so, as you can imagine, that wasn't fun. I now use a synthetic progestin, which I can tolerate well. It just took time to find what worked for me, and that could be true for you, too. That's why it's so important to find the right medical team and to speak up for yourself.

Remember, always put yourself first. If you feel that you're not being treated with the respect you deserve, look for a primary care doctor who is current on the latest studies and is willing to help you with your menopause symptoms.

WHEN MENOPAUSE AND MIDLIFE COLLIDE

Midway upon the journey of our life
I found myself within a forest dark
For the straightforward pathway had been lost.

DANTE'S *DIVINE COMEDY*

AVE YOU EVER googled the world "midlife"? The first thing that comes up is "midlife crisis," along with this definition at Wikipedia: "A midlife crisis is a transition of identity and self-confidence that can occur in middle-aged individuals, typically 45–64 years old." This just happens to coincide with the time women go through menopause.

I don't know about you, but I don't think that we should be identified as having a midlife crisis because of the symptoms and challenges of menopause. This term seems insensitive, as well as inaccurate, especially when a woman is having a particularly hard time with menopause or dealing with difficult major life events.

As we move into our forties and beyond, we face many challenges. We are no longer living the life that we did in our twenties and thirties (and in some cases, I say thank the Lord for that!). The challenges we faced back then fade into insignificance compared with the very real challenges we face right now.

In my twenties, the biggest decision I had to make was what outfit to buy from Top Shop for my Friday nights out. Now it's how to invest money for my kids' college funds while shouting at the neighborhood kids to get off my lawn. I mean, when did I become "that woman"? Seriously, life is just different now, and I'm completely fine with that. It's just that we face some challenges that we might not have expected: being an empty nester, making career decisions, or caring for elderly parents. This can be a difficult time in your life, especially with menopause thrown into the mix.

In Chapter 1, I discussed the potential physical and emotional symptoms menopause can bring. In addition to these symptoms, we are also dealing with perhaps the busiest and most hectic time in our lives, which can take an emotional toll on us.

There are so many life transitions that happen outside of the menopause shit-storm that digging deep into our coping skills becomes almost a daily requirement. When I added writing this book to my schedule I realized just how hectic my life is. In the beginning I committed to dedicating three solid hours to writing each day, so that I would stay on track and deliver the book on time. But normal life didn't just magically stop. I appear to have become an unpaid, unthanked Uber driver for my kids. Their crazy schedules have me creating such detailed calendars that I feel like their secretary. On top of this, I run an online

fitness company, and of course, I have my everyday obli-
gations to cook, do laundry, shop for food, clean the house,
help with homework, and be nice (sometimes that's the
most challenging). I'm pulled in so many different directions that finding enough time for myself, let alone to write
for three solid hours, became almost impossible.

I often found myself staring at a blank page wondering if it really was worth it to find thirty minutes to type
while the potatoes were boiling or asking myself if I should
bother my arse to research protein synthesis for the fifteen
minutes while I waited for my kids at the dentist. Already
feeling at maximum capacity, plus menopausing the crap
out of my life, I felt a whole new level of stress and disappointment during this writing process. I'm sure that many
of you feel equally stressed out.

One of the reasons midlife has been so closely associated
with crisis is that many women start to have feelings of
exhaustion, boredom, or unhappiness at this stage in their
life. Even if women are doing something that previously
gave them a sense of happiness and fulfillment, they might
feel the desire to try something new or different, but life
is just so busy that it seems impossible. Then throw in the
craziness of menopause, and it's no wonder that women
feel that they are permanently at war with themselves,
their life, and those around them. Might it be that you, too,
are simply trying to keep too many balls in the air?

FEAR

In addition to the many other symptoms that show up at
this time of life, many women start to feel more insecure,

with lower levels of self-esteem and belief in themselves and overwhelming feelings of vulnerability.

Five years ago, I was skiing down a moderately easy slope in British Columbia with my husband. We are both average-to-low-level skiers, so we generally stuck with the easy routes. Then suddenly he decided that we could veer off the run slightly and we came to what looked to me like a death drop. Ten years earlier I would have just taken a leap of faith and assumed I could make my way down, but on this day I froze. Then I had a mild anxiety episode: I freaked out.

To my husband's humiliation, I yanked off my skis, sat down on the snow, and slid the whole way down that big mountainside on my arse, the whole time screaming back to my husband that I would never forgive him for doing this to me and would never put skis on again. I didn't get back on skis for the rest of the holiday; I was just too scared. This was a new phenomenon for me, and I didn't like it. It was humiliating and utterly embarrassing.

Chapter 1 discussed the heightened anxiety that can occur during menopause because of declining sex hormones, and usually trotting right behind that is depression, with immense feelings of loss of hope. This is pretty much what happened to me on the ski slope: overwhelming anxiety followed by depression, feelings of disappointment, and lowered self-esteem. When did I stop being that fearless athlete ready to take on anything?

Fear and lack of belief in ourselves can also show up in our work. A career woman at the top of the corporate ladder may be feeling the pressures of work and home life, a woman whose career has stalled may fear changing direction, and a stay-at-home mother may feel the world is leaving her behind. How many times have you questioned whether what you're doing in your career is the right thing for you, for your family, and for your vision of success?

These challenges are real and can leave women at midlife feeling a huge sense of frustration, which is very stressful. It's worth taking the time to ask yourself where you are now in your life, whether you're happy there, and, if not, what you're going to do about it. I found myself in a void, not knowing what to do with my career. I enjoyed training clients in person, but my passion was dying.

It just so happened that I had to relocate two years ago and give up my in-person fitness business. This was an opportunity for me to try something else, but I knew I had limited skills for a new career and wasn't sure if I wanted to keep my fitness business at my new location. This period coincided with my deep depression, so the conditions for making such a decision were not ideal. In the end, even though I am still involved in the fitness business, writing articles and posting online workouts for my audience, I made the career decision to write this book.

INVISIBILITY

This is also the time of life when women can start to feel invisible. A few years ago, that idea made no sense to me. Then I started to experience it myself. All of a sudden it seemed that my voice was not being heard. There were a few occasions when I said something at the family table and the rest of the gang just carried on their conversation as though I hadn't spoken. Or another time, I said something that I felt was a good contribution with a group of peers, only to be completely ignored. Umm, hello, I'm still here. Did you even hear me speak? I felt like I'd started to fade into the background. The background is not a place I enjoy being, and I struggled to move forward from that position. It felt weird and annoying, and I knew I had to do something about it. I had to stop feeling invisible, but I also needed to find the energy to make a positive change.

There's a great article by Brené Brown called "The Midlife Unraveling." (Brené Brown lives in my town, and yet we have never had coffee together! How can this be?) In the article, Brené talks about her fight with the universe when faced with the crises that midlife was throwing at her. She says, "It was an ugly street fight and, even though I got my ass kicked, it was the best thing that ever happened to me. There was a significant amount of pain and loss, but something amazing happened along the way—I discovered me. The real me. The messy, imperfect, brave, scared, creative, loving, compassionate, wholehearted me."

That article made me realize that I had to start believing in myself again and standing up for what mattered. So that's what I did. I made myself comfortable in uncomfortable situations; I stepped out of the shadows.

I'm realizing more every day that my body is doing what it's naturally programmed to do, and my role is to support, protect, and love it. I'm not a victim, and I'm not broken. I feel pretty fierce, and the support here makes me feel powerful— I'm so ready to embrace what's next!

JENNIFER MCDOWELL EXOO, Menopausing So Hard member

LOSS OF SELF-ESTEEM

I am appalled that the term we use
to talk about aging is "anti." Aging is as natural
as a baby's softness and scent. Aging is human
evolution in its pure form.

JAMIE LEE CURTIS

Aging can be hard on a woman's feelings of worth and self-esteem. It's difficult for any woman over the age of thirty to feel good about herself if she uses images in the media as a measure of how she should look. I'm probably what's considered an old hag in the fitness industry, where the "ideal" representation of fitness is a nimble twenty-five-year-old in booty shorts. And I find it peculiar that although women over forty make up a large portion of gym goers, fitness magazines, websites, and social media never represent us. Instead we see ridiculous images of women who are starved within an inch of their lives, wrinkle-free, and cellulite-free, alongside articles telling us that we're too old or too fat or that we have too many wrinkles and saggy tits. Also, how dare you go gray! The cheek of it.

Well, I'm tired of all this codswallop. I'm tired of the way mainstream media chips away at the souls of older women, doing everything it can to point out our imperfections. It's no wonder some women grieve the loss of their youth and even the loss of their ability to get pregnant. The idea that their childbearing years are behind them can be a huge loss for many women. (A quick side note: my favorite hashtag is #aginghoweverthefuckyouwant. Your body, your business.)

To add insult to injury, we are constantly reminded of our lost youth by everybody else around us. At work we may feel that we aren't respected as much as our male counterparts—or if we are respected, then we have to work doubly hard to keep proving ourselves. At home we feel like constant failures if we don't live up to the pressures of being that perfect wife and mother. When my energy started waning in perimenopause, I felt as though I got nothing finished around the house. I don't know how many times I pulled together a list of excuses so I'd be ready when the hubby came home, explaining why I hardly got anything done—in fact, one day I actually wrote them down to justify my day (it was a long list, of course).

How sad and pathetic is that? And the kicker is that my husband didn't care. He knows I work hard, and he doesn't need to ask what I did all day as some sort of justification of my existence and worth.

But something quite amazing has happened to me in my forties. I've become okay with how my face is changing as I age. When I first started noticing those crinkles around my eyes in my thirties, I was horrified. I remember somebody sending me a photo, telling me it was their favorite photo of me, and I was gobsmacked. I couldn't stop fixating on how much my face had aged over that past decade and that people thought I looked "okay" like this. It really knocked my self-confidence, and I started looking at other women's faces, wondering how they felt about all that extra texture. Yet when I looked at the women who had influenced my life, that narrative didn't make sense to me. I never once judged them for aging—in fact, I admired that they did it with such grace.

Today I still see all the things I saw before, but now I'm okay with them. Now when I look at my face I see a person who has been through a shitty few years and emerged full of resilience and strength. I see somebody with passion, energy, history, stories, experience, and confidence. I have passed the phase in my life where I sweated the small stuff and have found a place of calm and fortitude. I give fewer fucks than I ever have and feel more alive than ever because of it.

So this is me and this is how it's going to be. Accepting where I am right now, being present and comfortable with aging, being brave enough to wear my wrinkles with pride. Ladies, when was the last time you looked at a raw photo of yourself and said, "I love this!"? I encourage you to try it.

———

I've dyed my hair since I was about fifteen. About two years ago—at age forty-nine—I decided I was fed up of touching up roots every three or four weeks and got my hairdresser to help me in the process of growing out the dye. So glad I did it . . . absolutely love my silver hair and now I can have some fun with pinks and purples.

BARBARA PARKINS,
Menopausing So Hard member

———

THE EMPTY NESTER

Menopause often coincides with becoming an empty nester. When children leave home, parents, and especially women, can be left with a feeling of loss and grief. "Empty nester syndrome" is not a clinical illness, but it can be a difficult transition period.

Children leaving home is the most natural occurrence in the world. We want them to go out into the big world and be independent. Yet it can sometimes leave women in particular feeling depressed and wondering what their purpose is now. Feelings of depression, anxiety, rejection, loss of purpose, and worry about their child's well-being can be overwhelming. These feelings are not a joke. Many women wrestle their way through this time, and if it coincides with menopause, they may have less ability to cope with stress. If feelings of loneliness and deep sadness take over, seek help from a medical professional.

On the flip side, if you're in this situation, this is a great opportunity to take a look at your life and make a special effort to take care of yourself. Many women use this as an opportunity to redefine their relationship with their children, to develop deeper connections with them on an entirely new, often more hands-off level, giving them the privacy and independence they need. It's wonderful to behold the child or children you helped develop into amazing adults. You should take huge pride in that.

This can also be a great opportunity to do things that interest you and to find new interests. Perhaps you've had an idea for a new career that you never had the time to invest in before, but now you can do it. New hobbies, traveling, social opportunities, a new career, and education are all possibilities that you could now have time to explore. It's time to overcome those feelings of fear and start to believe in yourself once again.

SQUEEZE GENERATION

Caring for two generations of family, one on either side of you, is common throughout midlife and can be overwhelming. On one side you have your children, who need you and depend on you, and on the other side you have elderly parents for whom you feel responsible. And what about you? Your career, your health, your relationship with your spouse or partner, and your sanity? There are only so many hours in the day, and with so many demands, you may already be stretched thin. Women typically take on too much, and we can often find it difficult to cope.

A 2009 survey by the National Alliance for Caregiving, in collaboration with the American Association of Retired Persons (AARP), found that an estimated 65.7 million people in the United States act as unpaid caregivers. The report determined that women are more likely than men to feel high stress. Half the caregivers surveyed said that their caregiving takes time away from friends and other family members and that they are far more likely to feel high emotional stress than those who have been able to maintain friends and family time.

Managing your stress should be a priority at any time in your life, but especially during menopause. The impact that stress can have on your health is huge. Caregiver burnout occurs when physical, emotional, and mental exhaustion takes hold and caregivers stop taking care of themselves, investing all of their energy into caring for ill or elderly loved ones. They may do this out of a sense of duty or guilt, and the body can only cope with so much; if we don't accept enough help from others, there's a danger that chronic stress will take over.

CHANGING RELATIONSHIPS

I once flippantly told a friend that I bet most divorces happen during menopause. We can't cope with the shit we used to put up with before, because we're stressed, hormonal, maybe depressed, and riddled with anxiety. We may be contemplating new beginnings, careers, and life choices—so why wouldn't we contemplate getting rid of the husband? I said it in jest, but when I was at my lowest with depression, I *did* wonder if it was because I was unhappy in my marriage. This was a passing thought, but still, I really had to dig deep to find the positives that existed between my husband and me. They had always been there, but my depression was clouding reality.

That got me wondering: *Do* more divorces happen during menopause? The AARP says that more than 60 percent of divorces are initiated by women in their forties, fifties, and sixties—that is, our menopause years. So why is this happening?

I hate the way we blame our hormones for everything, but it really is worth pondering here. When our levels of estrogen drop, so does our level of oxytocin. Oxytocin is one of our feel-good hormones; it reduces our inhibitions in social encounters and reduces our anxieties. It's sometimes referred to as the "love hormone," sending messages to the brain especially during sex, birth, and breastfeeding—it helps us bond with our partners and our children. Oxytocin has also been shown to be an antidote to depressive feelings and to affect our orgasms (more on that in Chapter 4).

So what have estrogen and oxytocin got to do with divorce? Some doctors think that this drop in oxytocin can change the female way of thinking from the "we" mindset to the "me" mindset, and men don't like that. Can you imagine starting to put ourselves first for a change? I see this all the time: it's like a light-bulb moment for women to realize that they can, in fact, make a decision that affects themselves first, over others.

It's time to stop placing the blame on ourselves, ladies. We are going through an evolutionary process with our bodies that means stuff is going to change. Our view of relationships is just one example. Speaking with your partner, being open about what you're experiencing, how you're coping, and what help you need will really help your partner understand. In fact, why not get them to read this book? This can also be a time to redefine what your marriage or partnership is.

My husband was blindsided by my menopause experience, which left him feeling isolated and confused. I barely had an understanding of what was happening, so there was little chance that he was going to understand. I realized that I needed to create a different environment for us to be closer and a new dialogue between us that would keep us emotionally connected.

It's brought my partner and me closer together.
He didn't understand female bodies before but he
sure does now. The heavy periods, the night sweats,
the forgetfulness, the weight gain. We've strength-
ened our team to where we can tackle anything
and everything together.

KARI BROWN, Menopausing So Hard member

THE POSITIVE STUFF

When faced with the menopause shit-storm, it's no wonder we are often left feeling like some whack-job crazy bitch who has lost control of life. But an amazing thing can happen when you let menopause in, when you accept that it's happening (once you understand that it is really happening)—it's almost magical. We tend to identify with something more positively when we can name it. Once you have labeled yourself as going through menopause, you can start making some mental and physical shifts to forge through it, and you can be quite creative and ingenious in your methods.

Studies show quite clearly that our positivity and outlook on life follow a U-shaped curve, dropping somewhat in midlife and improving drastically as we age. Laura L. Carstensen, a professor of psychology at Stanford University, studies longevity and has produced numerous publications showing that our satisfaction with life improves from our mid-fifties until our seventies, when it peaks. We may be in the bottom of the U right now, but there's a glimmer of light at the top of the curve and we have to keep pushing toward it.

Focusing on the positives can help manage your stress levels, improve your relationships, ease some of the burdens you place on yourself, and give you the freedom to enjoy life, whatever that might look like to you.

Just for shits and giggles, I asked myself about the positive aspects of menopause, and I realized there were many—despite everything I had experienced and continue to experience. For starters, my periods are over, which is a huge money-saver and convenience. I hardly have any hair growing on my body anymore, and I love that I barely need to shave my legs or underarms (though I am concerned about getting a hairy face; I'm not sure how positive I'll feel if I start to look like Nanny McPhee!). During perimenopause, as my hormones fluctuated, my boobs actually got bigger; well, truthfully, this was not a positive for me, but it was for my husband.

Lastly and more seriously, an amazing sense of calm has descended on me. It took its time arriving, but now it is here and I feel so much happier. The ability to stop sweating the small stuff feels like a gift from the gods. I have developed more patience with and empathy for my children's anxieties and troubles. Now it looks as though I actually give a shit (which I do) and I also look like an amazing mother (which maybe I am!).

My relationship with my husband is just different. It's still sexy and fun, but it's also more loving, more caring, and fuller; we do more together, we have more adventures, we want to create more memories.

There are positives out there if you just allow yourself to find them. You can be the aggressor toward menopause or you can be the peacemaker.

— 4 —

HELLO, DRY VAGINA AND INCONTINENCE

YOU'VE PROBABLY REALIZED by now that there are very few boundaries in my work. I want to talk about all aspects of menopause openly, and that includes all the juicy goodness about your Queen V.

Menopause can do a number on your vagina and related parts, leaving many of you struggling with erratic periods, vaginal dryness, strange smells, incontinence, and painful sex.

As if that weren't enough to dampen your sex life, shifting hormone levels also step in to hammer your libido. Do you ever look around for your mojo and wonder where the heck it went? Mine got up and disappeared for a while. But don't worry, you aren't alone, it's a pretty normal thing to experience, and there are things you can do to get it back. Phew!!

I was cursed with every one of the ailments mentioned above. None of it was expected and all of it was confusing. But after extensive reading and conversations with many women, I realize that it's all part of the rite of passage. If you feel that any of your symptoms are extreme, however, or if you're worried about them, then take yourself along to your health care provider and get a thorough checkup.

IRREGULAR PERIODS AND THE ALIEN BIRTH

One of my favorite games to play is period roulette. When you start spotting and then nothing happens . . . the thrill of not knowing how this is going to go just never, ever gets old. Alienbaby period? Regular? Or nothing? And then there's the adrenaline rush from stacking your purse with a wide range of products and extra underwear just to be ready for all scenarios. It's like a different version of survival.

ANNE BELL,
Menopausing So Hard member

Your hormones are irregular in perimenopause; therefore your menstrual cycle probably will be as well. Some women never see a change in their cycle throughout the whole of perimenopause; it just tapers off toward menopause. But most women find that their periods become somewhat or very erratic. When this happens it's hard to plan for. My advice for the whole of perimenopause, and that could be ten years, is don't wear white trousers! Seriously, WTF! It can be really frustrating, especially if your normal PMS symptoms have changed and you have no idea when your next period will show up. Your menopause tracker can come in handy in keeping track of your cycle. Even if there isn't an obvious pattern, there may be some familiar symptoms that will give you a heads-up to keep some extra tampons in your bag.

Your periods might start getting lighter. You might get spotting mid-cycle, and at other times you might feel as though you're birthing a whole alien—I once had a period so heavy, with clumps of "stuff" being evacuated (I told you there were no boundaries in this chapter), that I had to change my tampon hourly for a whole day. Eventually, when the heavy bleeding subsided, I continued to bleed for more than thirty days. It was crazy. During that time, I felt completely healthy, and the bleeding, although heavy, felt normal too. Some women do get severe bleeding that must be checked out, so please go to a doctor if you're concerned.

I actually assumed that the mass exodus of blood was the final salute from my ovaries. Unfortunately, that was not the case, and I continued to have very light periods every seven months for a couple of years.

My best advice is to be prepared for the unexpected. Carry sanitary products with you permanently. I took to using a menstrual cup, which is a small plastic cup you insert in your vagina during periods; it's a little more environmentally friendly than a tampon and also easy to keep in your purse. Take to wearing a daily sanitary pad, darker clothes, or underwear that's purposely made for periods, like Thinx, which absorbs bleeding into the fabric.

HORMONES AND SMELLS

There are some days when I really smell bad. Yes, I stink! I really do. My armpits can smell like a dirty old jock-strap. I have never stunk like this before. So many things could be contributing to this change in body odor. When you ovulate, you release more of a "male" smell, and as your hormone levels become more erratic, the smell may worsen. Hormonal fluctuations can cause hot flashes and night sweats, and increased anxiety can also make you struggle with lovely, stinky B.O. If excessive sweating and increased body odor starts to have an impact on your life, then speak to your doctor, as there are some medications available to control this.

You may also notice a change in the smell of your vagina. As your estrogen levels drop, your vag will start to dry out and your secretions will lessen. The drop in hormones also causes your pH levels to change, which can cause a slightly unpleasant odor. On occasion, down in the nether regions, I am certain that I detect a stale old-lady odor, which is just so gross. In my menopause community, we have unanimously decided we reek of "pickled skunk."

Finally, some women struggle with incontinence, and a few dribbles here and there can leave an unpleasant scent.

The good news is that the smells begin to ease as your hormones start to calm down. In the meantime there are a few ways you can manage these odors:

- Wash with water but not soap to ensure that you don't alter the delicate pH level of your vagina. A cleanser like Cerave Hydrating Cleanser is a great alternative. It's not necessary or often safe to invest in feminine hygiene washes.

- Manage your stress levels. This is funny, right? But try some of the stress-management tips in Chapter 9.

- If the odors become chronic (long-lasting), visit your doctor.

- If the odor is accompanied by pain or itching, see a doctor immediately.

But remember: your vag isn't supposed to smell like a bloody rose garden, so don't fall for a marketing spiel that tells you otherwise.

VAGINAL ATROPHY/GENITOURINARY SYNDROME OF MENOPAUSE (GSM)

Another surprise that menopause gifts us is vaginal atrophy, which is when the tissues of the vulva and vagina become more fragile because of menopause. I am not that fond of the term "atrophy," and it doesn't accurately describe what happens when estrogen levels decline. Because vaginal atrophy often includes urinary symptoms, it's now referred to as genitourinary syndrome of menopause (GSM). In her 2019 book *The Vagina Bible*, Dr. Jen Gunter explains that "while the lower third of the vagina and vestibule (vaginal opening) are rich with estrogen receptors and consequently can be significantly impacted by menopause, there are estrogen receptors in the clitoris, labia, urethra, and bladder, and so the symptoms and physical changes are not confined to the vagina."

As estrogen declines, your body's tissues lose collagen and therefore elasticity (hence my extra facial wrinkles) and the lining of your uterus can start to thin. The basic integrity of the vagina starts to degrade, and you may experience thinning of the vaginal walls, some inflammation, and dryness. Women often find these changes very embarrassing and painful. Other symptoms of GSM include incontinence, bacterial vaginitis, and urinary tract infections, as well as burning, itching, discharge, tearing of skin, and spotting of blood.

Because the vaginal wall can become so fragile, it may tear or bleed during sex, which can cause pain and discomfort. Small wonder that women feel like they should stop having penetrative sex, either with their partner or with a vibrator.

Dr. Lauren Streicher is on a mission to change sandpaper sex into slippery sex. You have to love a woman with that as her mission. More than 50 percent of postmenopausal women suffer from vaginal issues as a result of GSM, yet only 7 percent do anything about it. Most simply put up with the pain or give up on sex.

Many women don't seek out treatment, suffering in silence, when this isn't necessary. This might be due to the delicate nature of the problem or they might think they'll be dismissed or misdiagnosed. Adopting good hygiene and working with a medical provider are essential to treating GSM. Let's look at some of the options.

- *Topical estrogen creams.* Your doctor might suggest trying estrogen cream to restore some vitality to your vagina. Studies have shown improvement of GSM symptoms in menopausal women who use estrogen cream.

Estrogen cream stays localized in the vagina and can often be an option for those who can't take HT because of breast cancer. According to the ACOG, data does not show an increased risk of cancer recurrence among women currently undergoing treatment for breast cancer or those with a personal history of breast cancer who use vaginal estrogen to relieve urogenital symptoms. Talk to your doctor about whether this is a viable option for you.

- *Lubricants.* These are used primarily before sex to create a slippery passage. They do not change or improve the integrity of your vagina. You can get water-based or silicone-based, both of which work fine, but look for a brand that's pH balanced (vaginal pH is acidic, typically with a pH of 3.8 to 4.5), which won't dry you out too much.

- *Vaginal moisturizers.* Only one product, Replens, has been proven in scientific studies to thicken vaginal walls, increase lubrication, and decrease painful intercourse. It should be applied daily. It can be applied two hours before having intercourse, which allows proper moisturization.

- *Laser treatment.* Laser treatments are now available for vaginal rejuvenation. Laser treatment is a relatively painless and simple procedure and is used as an alternative to hormonal treatment. But it does come with a word of warning from Dr. Stephanie Faubion, medical director for NAMS: "Although vaginal laser therapy for treatment of GSM is promising, data are still lacking regarding long-term safety and efficacy using well-designed placebo-controlled studies." Ask your doctor about it, but be prepared to spend big bucks.

- *DHEA vaginal inserts.* This is an FDA-approved non-estrogen treatment called Intrarosa that has been clinically proven to mitigate painful sex and improve the vaginal tissue. DHEA is a precursor steroid hormone produced mainly in the adrenal glands. DHEA naturally declines with age, but can be an important source of estrogen and testosterone for women. Once inserted vaginally, Intrarosa converts to estrogen and testosterone, although the mechanism of the action of Intrarosa is not fully understood. For what it's worth, I have used this treatment intermittently and found it to be very helpful.

- *HT.* As discussed in Chapter 2, HT taken orally or transdermally puts estrogen back into your system. Sometimes HT is enough to make GSM manageable. I struggled terribly with incontinence, dryness, painful sex, and bacterial vaginitis, and all of those completely went away when I started HT.

URINARY INCONTINENCE

I spoke candidly about my incontinence issues in Chapter 1. If this is an issue for you, I highly recommend finding a pelvic-floor physiotherapist who will guide you in an exercise program to help strengthen your whole pelvic-floor region. What I didn't tell you was that a month or so after working with my pelvic-floor physio, I peed my pants again. Or should I say I peezed, a combination of sneezing and peeing at the same time, the ultimate multitasking.

I was still doing my pelvic-floor exercises regularly, so something else was clearly amiss. I went to my gynecologist, who told me that some women find that incontinence can come and go as hormones fluctuate. Whenever I went through a period of incontinence, I entered it into my menopause tracker. It became clear to me that in addition to maintaining my pelvic-floor health with exercises, I also needed to be aware that the incontinence would come and go as my hormones continued to be erratic. After starting HT, however, I didn't have any more incontinence issues.

This was a very frustrating experience and yet another thing I wasn't expecting. I initially struggled to find out why it was happening, and I got very annoyed when people advised me to simply do more Kegels. I wanted to know what was going on, not simply be given a solution that might or might not have been relevant to me.

Falling levels of estrogen can cause thinning in the lining of the urethra (our pee tube, taking urine from the bladder out of the body), in addition to weakening of the pelvic floor, which can cause incontinence.

Up to 45 percent of women will suffer from urinary incontinence during their lifetime. This problem is very common but it's not normal, and it can be treated, so find a good health care provider and physiotherapist who can help you with this complex problem.

Incontinence shows up in a few different ways, so it is helpful to identify what type of incontinence you are experiencing.

Stress urinary incontinence is caused by intra-abdominal pressure, which occurs when you cough, sneeze, run, jump rope, or perform some other strenuous exercise. In my example, peezing is the ultimate SUI.

Urge urinary incontinence, as you might imagine, is associated with urgency. For example, when you're trying to get the key in the front door of the house so that you can go to the bathroom but don't think you can make it. Sometimes even hearing the sound of running water can cause you to have leakage.

Lastly, there's mixed urinary incontinence, in which you suffer from both stress urinary incontinence and urge urinary incontinence.

Whatever kind of incontinence you might have, don't give up hope. There are things you can do to stop those leaks:

- Seek out a pelvic-floor physiotherapist.

- Control your weight. Obesity is a strong independent factor for incontinence.

- Anxiety and stress have been associated with incontinence, so try adopting stress-management techniques (see breathing, below).

- Retrain your pelvic floor with daily Kegel exercises (see below).

- Speak to your doctor about HT and/or topical estrogen cream, which has been shown to improve incontinence.

Surgery is another option, but it should be considered only after you have exhausted all other options and have discussed it with your doctor.

UTIs (URINARY TRACT INFECTIONS)

I experienced my first ever UTI this year, and it made me feel incredibly ill. I initially thought I had food poisoning, because I couldn't stop puking. The next day when I had to nip to the loo for the tenth time, I realized that I might have a UTI. A quick pee stick purchased from Walmart confirmed this so I headed to the doctor. Boy, did I feel rotten, but within a few days of taking antibiotics I was totally fine again.

More than three million women suffer from UTIs annually, and they are very common during menopause. So why does this keep happening? Well, our vaginas are inhabited by lots of healthy bacteria which happily co-exist, with estrogen allowing good bacteria called Lactobacillus to thrive. This bacteria produces acid which then lowers the pH levels in our vagina, keeping the bad bacteria out. You following? As we know in menopause, estrogen declines and that in turn alters the level of good bacteria and acid in the vagina, making it easier for the unwanted bacteria to be absorbed. Infections can occur when the usually sterile urinary tract (where pee comes from) gets infiltrated by bacteria from either the nearby rectum or the vagina and voila, you have a UTI. I must point out, though, that there is absolutely no evidence to suggest that UTIs are a result of uncleanliness; it's more about the level of acidity and its role with bacteria. It sucks big time, but menopause can mean that you're just going to be more susceptible to them.

Some signs of a UTI are increased frequency and urgency to pee, darker urine, and painful burning sensations when you pee. You may also have lower back or abdomen pain, overall fatigue, and fever.

You must see a doctor and get on antibiotics if this happens. Your doctor will diagnose your UTI by your symptoms and a urine culture test.

Preventively there are a few things you can do:

- *Cranberry extract.* There is no evidence to suggest that cranberry juice helps with UTIs, plus it's loaded with added sugar. Some studies have shown that cranberry extract in tablet form may help prevent the bad bacteria from sticking to vaginal walls, but these are low-quality studies. It seems that you would have to take high levels of cranberry for it to be effective, and the supplements are not regulated. My advice is to take them if your doctor suggests it after diagnosis, in addition to the antibiotics that will be prescribed, and don't completely give up on the idea that they might be helpful.

- *Peeing properly.* Adopt healthy urinary habits:

  › Don't strain or push to pee; relax as much as possible, and let the urine flow.

  › Be patient and let the bladder empty completely.

- *Vaginal estrogen creams/inserts.* These can help restore the natural balance of bacteria in your vagina if you are constantly having episodes.

- *Drink water.* Staying hydrated and peeing frequently help the body flush out unwanted bacteria. In general, holding in urine and not emptying your bladder fully can increase your likelihood of getting an infection.

If you are struggling with frequent UTIs, speak to your doctor about taking an antibiotic prophylactically.

PELVIC-FLOOR HEALTH
AND KEGELS DONE RIGHT

A woman's pelvic floor consists of muscles, ligaments, connective tissues, and nerves that support the bladder, uterus, vagina, and rectum and help these pelvic organs to function. Fluctuating hormones affect the pelvic floor's function and strength, however.

Adopting habits that keep your pelvic floor healthy is something I recommend to all women, regardless of whether you have gone through pregnancy or not. During menopause, the structure of your pelvic-floor muscles is going to change. As I have mentioned, some women may experience incontinence; others may have a uterine prolapse, where the pelvic floor stretches and weakens enough that the uterus is no longer supported, and it protrudes into the vagina.

There are a few strategies that you can start practicing to strengthen your pelvic floor. These include correcting your posture, controlling your core, and practicing breathing exercises and Kegels (which must be done the right way). My intention is to simplify all of this information so that it is easy to incorporate into your daily life.

The importance of posture is often undersold in the fitness industry because it's not sexy and a little bit boring. But by improving your posture you can prevent injuries and ailments, including a leaky pelvic floor. Then, by building strength and stability throughout your core, you can exercise in a position that's both safe and effective. I'm a little bit of a drill sergeant when it comes to exercise, and that's because I know how important it is to create a stable, injury-free body as we age.

I'm sure you've heard people being told to stand up straight, pull their shoulders back, suck in their belly—all cues that force us to stand tall and straight. What annoys me about those cues is that they create a ton of tension in your body and make you feel uncomfortable, which is the opposite of what you need to do to have a solid posture. Good posture is going to look different on every person, but there are some key areas that you need to be aware of to find yours.

If you don't have a good posture, it will often present itself in a number of ways:

- Posterior pelvic tilt, where your bottom is tucked under

- Ribcage flared out or shifted backward, which means the core has a hard time developing any stability

- Flattened lower back, with glutes that are not engaged, again preventing the body from attaining enough tone and strength throughout the core

- Anterior pelvic tilt, which sometimes occurs during exercise, where the bottom sticks out and the lower back is hyperextended

HOW TO CORRECT YOUR POSTURE

This might take you a little while to understand, so I like to suggest standing in front of a mirror to help you both see and feel what it's like to have good posture. It might feel awkward and unnatural at first, but please persist!

Stand up tall and be as relaxed as possible before you start this exercise. Understand that this might take time to practice and that during the day it's a good idea to recheck your posture and correct it. I advise my clients to do this after they wash their hands when they pee. Over time, this constant practice will pay off, and your body will start to understand what good alignment is.

- Reach tall through the crown of your head and lengthen your spine.

- Now check your ribs at the front of your body. Are they sticking out in front of you? Place your hands on your ribs and push down; this will tuck those ribs back in so you can feel them meet your stomach.

- Is your bum sticking out? Your lower back will likely have a natural small arch in it, which is good, but make sure you do not intentionally stick your bum out or actively tuck it underneath you.

- Let your arms hang down by your sides and then externally rotate them so that your inside elbow creases are facing forward. This has the wonderful effect of putting the shoulders in a great position.

The result is that your shoulders, ribs, and hips should all be stacked nicely on top of one another.

HOW TO CONTROL YOUR CORE

When I talk about your core, I'm not referring to your six-pack or the front line of your body. There is a misconception that the core is the "abs"—unfortunately, fitness vanity has led us down that path. The core is actually a little more complex than that, and basically includes anything front and back located between your shoulders and hips—your trunk, essentially. Your core is made up of four muscles, which are critical to the functioning of your pelvic floor.

Think of your core as a cube made up of the following muscles:

- diaphragm (top)

- pelvic floor (bottom)

- deep abdominal muscle (transversus abdominis, or TVA) (front)

- lower back muscle (multifidus—a very long and thin muscle deep in the spine) (back)

These four muscle groups work together as a team. They rely on one another to function optimally so that your core is strong and stable. Because they work in unison, if one of those muscle groups isn't working optimally, you might see a weakness, which often shows up as a sore lower back, tight shoulders, or pelvic-floor issues such as incontinence and prolapse.

Diaphragm. This is a dome-shaped muscle that sits at the top of the core. It is located under our ribs and is our primary breathing muscle. The muscle is attached to both the rib cage and the lower back vertebrae, which makes the diaphragm an important postural muscle as well as a respiratory one. In addition, the diaphragm runs through our hip flexor muscle (the psoas), which is the only muscle that connects our spine with our legs. Sometimes lower back pain and tight hips can be associated with diaphragm restrictions, so deep-breathing exercises can be beneficial.

Pelvic floor. This consists of a series of muscles and tissues that stretch from your tailbone all the way forward to your pubic bone. Imagine a sling or a hammock that holds in your bladder, uterus, and bowels. When the integrity of the pelvic floor is weakened or fragile, you can see how this might cause you problems. Because they are a group of muscles, you can exercise them to function correctly and strengthen over time—and it's important to do so.

TVA and lower back. This group of muscles creates the front and back of the core. If you struggle with lower back issues, a weak core, or diastasis rectus—a condition caused after pregnancy where your abs don't close back up—you might struggle to develop total control over the whole core area. Building up strength throughout the whole trunk can help you gain control of your pelvic floor.

Now that you are aware of what the core consists of, let's look at how breathing plays a big part in activating these muscles.

HOW TO BREATHE FOR PELVIC-FLOOR HEALTH

I've talked about how important posture is for overall body health, and this—combined with understanding breathing mechanics—is the killer key to strengthening your pelvic-floor muscles. Good alignment allows the spine and the rib cage to position themselves so that the diaphragm moves optimally. And remember, the diaphragm works with the pelvic floor as a team, so working on the diaphragmatic breath is an easy way to stabilize that area and strengthen any weaknesses there.

If when you breathe you feel your shoulders lifting— rather than your ribs pushing out to the side and your belly getting big—then you are likely using your upper chest area rather than the diaphragm. Chest breaths are shallow; you will feel the breath more in your upper back and neck. Have upper body tension? This is probably why.

The following breathing technique, called box-breathing or four-square breathing, comes from years of practicing yoga in my thirties, and it's so easy to perform that it's my go-to exercise. It is also a great way to reduce stress and anxiety.

To start: Sit in an upright, comfortable chair, feet flat on the floor. Sitting up as straight as you can, try to focus on your posture. When you're ready, start with step 1.

Step 1: Inhale

Inhale through your nose for a slow count of four. Be aware of the process; do this consciously. The air should first fill your lungs until they're completely full and then start to fill your belly so that you end up looking like Buddha.

Step 2: Hold

Hold your breath for another slow count of four.

Step 3: Exhale

Breathe out, through your nose or your mouth, for another slow count of four, until both your belly and chest are completely empty. You may feel a slight contraction on your abs as you do this.

Step 4: Hold
Hold your breath for the same slow count of four.

Step 5: Repeat
Repeat the whole process two or three times in total.

All in all, this should only take you two or three minutes each time. Ideally you should practice this daily.

Now that you know how to breathe consciously, maybe you would like to know why it helps your pelvic-floor health? As I mentioned earlier, your core muscles work as a team. So by focusing on breathing, you will expand and contract your diaphragm. Every breath you take (cue Sting) gives you the opportunity to improve the strength and function of your pelvic floor.

When you breathe in, the diaphragm contracts (gets smaller) and allows you to breathe deeply into the belly, and the pelvic floor, TVA, and multifidus all relax. If you just inhale now, focus on your pelvic floor and feel it expand and soften and completely relax.

When you breathe out, the diaphragm relaxes back up to its original position and the pelvic floor contracts; you might feel it lift up. As you continue to exhale, your multifidus and TVA will also contract, and you might feel your abs engage.

KEGELS DONE PROPERLY!

Now that you have good posture and have mastered breathing to help your core function correctly, let's talk about Kegels. Kegels have been bastardized over the years. I remember my doctor telling me to go home and practice Kegels by clenching my pelvic-floor muscles really hard and holding that position ten times each day. Unfortunately, all that is doing is creating more tension in your nether regions.

I have just shown you how breathing can help you release tension so that your pelvic floor can contract and expand naturally rather than in a forced fashion, and that's also how you need to practice your Kegels. Over the years I've learned many cues that can help explain how to perform a Kegel, but I think my favorite is from pelvic-floor expert Julie Wiebe.

Sitting on a hard surface or in an upright chair, take a deep breath into your belly, as in box-breathing, and relax your body completely. Then, on the exhale, imagine pulling a Kleenex out of a box. The opening of the Kleenex box is the opening of your vagina, and you're pulling the pelvic-floor muscles up to lift out the Kleenex.

PUTTING IT ALL TOGETHER

Now, because the body works as a combined system, isolating your pelvic floor and doing Kegel exercises are not likely to help you very much with incontinence. You need to integrate your Kegels with your posture and breathing for maximum effect.

Let's pull all that together.

In this easy three-step process, you will not only sort out your postural issues but also learn to use breathing to help with Kegel exercises for pelvic-floor health.

Step 1. Remember your posture cues.

Step 2. Practice box-breathing.

Step 3. Integrate Kegel exercises.

Here's how!

This complete breathing exercise will help to relax the muscles of your pelvic floor, where you might hold tension, and to retrain your inner-core muscles to provide support. This is about allowing your body to function correctly rather than forcing it to do so. Make sure you tune into your breath throughout, feeling it coming into and then leaving your body.

- Sit on a hard chair or bench and stack your shoulders, ribs and hips (posture cue).

- Inhale for a count of four, focusing on inflating and relaxing the pelvic floor onto the chair.

- Hold your breath for a count of four.

- Exhale for a count of four, focusing on lifting your vagina and anus up and into your body. Remember the Kleenex cue: gently lift it out of the box for the full count of four. This is not an aggressive action—use around 30 percent of your maximum effort. At the end of the exhale, you will feel your abs contract slightly.

- Hold your breath for a count of four.

- Repeat two to three times in total.

- Do this five to seven times a week.

Posture + Breathing + Kegels = A healthy pelvic floor

If you are concerned about the time required for you to do this on top of all the other things you're doing, bear in mind that it will take around four minutes to complete this in total. You could do this at your desk at work or watching telly with your loved ones. It takes practice and at first feels very strange, but I promise you this sort of exercise is going to be invaluable to you—especially as you age, when many women experience incontinence and other pelvic-floor issues.

I ENCOURAGE YOU to talk with your doctor about all of these issues. Remember, there's nothing to be ashamed of. I am so over feeling embarrassed by these issues, and you should be too. Advocate for yourself and don't be afraid to ask for second opinions or alternatives to treatments offered to you. There is no reason for you to suffer from these problems during menopause.

— 5 —

I'M SO BLOODY FAT!

I F I HAD a dollar for every time a menopausal woman asked me how to lose her menopause belly, I'd be a millionaire!

The statistics aren't great, according to Dr. Amos Pines, former president of the International Menopause Society, who says that nine out of ten American women will gain weight during menopause. Around the world, that number is around 70 percent. Women who believe they haven't changed anything in their diet or their exercise routine suddenly pile on the pounds and it doesn't seem to make sense, which can be frustrating and demoralizing.

I have always been the classic pear-shaped lady, all bum and legs. I never put on weight on my tummy—in fact, I rocked a six-pack for most of my thirties and into my early forties. When I entered perimenopause and my symptoms seemed borderline aggressive, my weight stayed the same, but my body started to change shape. I started to notice that my tum-tum was a wee bit softer and rounder than before, my boobs had exploded in size, and I had been hit with the dreaded "back fat"! Yes, my body was now draped in the menopause flesh cloak.

A few years into perimenopause, I jumped on the scales and found that my weight had increased by ten pounds. That isn't so bad, but my body had started to look unrecognizable to me (i.e., the only person that mattered). Like many women, I felt confused and, truthfully, somewhat embarrassed by my new shape, especially when my clothes didn't fit properly anymore.

Funnily enough, the hardest thing for me to wrap my head around was gaining weight in my boobs. I always loved having a small, boy-like chest that meant I didn't really need to wear a bra and my boobs never got in the way when I was exercising. During pregnancy my bra size grew to 36DD, but afterward I went back to my former size quite rapidly.

When I was in perimenopause with my yo-yoing hormones, my boobs jumped from two hanging pieces of tissue resembling eggs in a pair of stockings to these huge masses of flesh that reminded me of cow udders. In fact, one day at the movies while in my cow-udder phase, I lost an earring—and found it two days later, underneath the fold of my left boob. Ew, so gross.

I have spent more than two decades coaching women to respect and honor their bodies. I've instilled the message that the number on the scale doesn't define them and that a few extra pounds does not make them any less of a person or any less attractive. I never judge a woman on the size or shape of her body, and my job as a coach is to help women feel the same way about themselves.

So although initially I did feel a little embarrassed by my weight gain, I was quick to pull from my own coaching. Instead of dwelling on those few extra pounds, I decided to use this as an opportunity to find out exactly why it had happened through honest reflection on my own habits, conversations with other women, and digging deep into the research. The symptomatic side of menopause had been nothing short of hell. On reflection I knew I wasn't exercising consistently, I was eating too much, and I was stressed up to my eyeballs. These are all contributing factors to putting on weight, and it had crept up on me slowly while I was knee-deep in symptoms. It took me a while to feel comfortable with the little extra softness and curves, as I had always been afraid of getting bigger or seeing the number on my scale increase. I still wanted to lose that ten pounds, or at least some of it, but I decided that I was going to be cool with my new look and stop feeling embarrassed by a few extra pounds.

I am using my weight gain as an example to show how I had to change my attitude and view of myself—but come on, ten pounds is nothing. Many women I speak to gain much more than ten pounds, and self-acceptance is much more difficult. When you've put on twenty, thirty, or forty-plus pounds, it can be really difficult to get that ugly thought monster telling you that you're worthless out of your head. Yet that's a very important part of the process, and gaining control of your health must start there.

I often make jokes and try to put things in a lighter shade, but that doesn't mean I don't understand the huge impact that weight gain and changes in body shape during menopause can have. As you might expect, there isn't one single answer to the burning question of weight gain. It's multilayered. Let's look at what we know about weight gain in menopause and what we can do about it.

WHAT WE KNOW ABOUT WEIGHT GAIN

Why do many women gain weight during menopause? There is rarely a single reason why anyone gains weight. We need to take several factors into consideration, and that's just as true in menopause as during other times in our lives. At the same time, there seems to be something about menopause that makes it even easier to gain weight and makes losing weight seem like a complete impossibility.

Crushing symptoms can make it hard to prioritize things like regular exercise and making good nutritional choices. We live high-stress lives that are detrimental to our well-being, and all of these factors can lead to weight gain.

It is possible to lose weight during menopause, and it simply isn't true that your menopause potbelly is here to stay. Hormonal changes directly affect the way your body copes with food, stress, and other lifestyle factors. Therefore, everything you do must also change. The old ways won't work anymore. I lost most of that naughty ten pounds that crept up on me, and I have helped many women get back to a healthy weight by focusing in new ways on the areas that we can positively affect, like nutrition, exercise, stress management, and positive mindset as we age.

In this chapter I explore some of the hurdles you are up against in dealing with menopausal weight gain, which include the cortisol and insulin connection, your hunger hormones, increased adipose tissue, bloating and water retention, and, finally, how we look at weight gain as a negative thing.

THE CORTISOL AND INSULIN CONNECTION

Cortisol is a steroid hormone produced in our adrenal glands (near our kidneys), and it is necessary for our well-being. It often gets a bad rap, but it actually serves a purpose. Cortisol is released in response to stress and it prompts glucose to be released into the body for energy. Imagine a saber-tooth tiger running at you; if you don't run fast, you're going to get eaten alive. Cortisol is what will save your life, giving you the ability to access glucose and run really fast.

You don't need to be chased down by a prehistoric animal to release cortisol, however. It is also released in everyday stressful situations, such as a bad day at the office. It is also released in short bursts during exercise, which is considered a stressor on your body.

In order for glucose to be released, the body has to suppress insulin, a hormone produced in your pancreas every time you eat. Insulin enables your body to use the sugar in the carbs you eat, which breaks down in the bloodstream as glucose. Insulin's job is to carry that glucose to the muscles, liver, or fat cells, where it is stored, ready to be used as energy and reducing the glucose in the bloodstream.

Are you still following along?

The following scenario shows how cortisol and insulin are connected:

- You're faced with a stressful situation: your boss wants you to stay at work until 8:00 PM, but you have to get home for the kids.

- Your body releases cortisol in response to this stressor. Your heart rate increases and the blood starts pumping (and your head is about to pop off!).

- Cortisol's job is to prepare your body for fight-or-flight by releasing glucose, mainly from the liver, giving you instant energy (this is your chance to become a superhero).

- Cortisol then inhibits insulin production, because you need that glucose availability *now*!

- When you resolve this head-popping situation by taking a deep breath and deciding to complete your work at home so that you can be with the kids, your insulin and cortisol levels return to normal levels.

In menopause, low estrogen affects your ability to cope with stress. If you're constantly in a heightened state of stress, you produce more cortisol and likely become less insulin-sensitive, meaning you churn out more insulin than you need, leading to weight gain, especially in the belly.

Cortisol and insulin are hormones that are fortunately under our control, whereas estrogen and progesterone must decline in order for us to reach menopause.

HT has been shown to help with the erratic nature of cortisol and insulin. Here are some other steps you can take to lessen the impact of these hormones.

Cortisol is a response to stressors, which can be wide-ranging and include insomnia, hot flashes, migraines, too much alcohol, smoking, poor diet, and work and life challenges. You therefore need to introduce protocols to manage your stress. Great lifestyle choices you can make include regular exercise, a balanced diet, and stress-management techniques such as sleep hygiene, meditation, yoga, and walking. All have been shown to improve quality of life and longevity. Stress is covered in more detail in Chapter 9.

You can also control insulin, using similar protocols to those for cortisol and making long-lasting changes in your lifestyle. Improving your diet, along with introducing resistance training and stress-management techniques, will result in improved insulin response; this is covered in more detail in Part 2.

HUNGER HORMONES

Are you hungry all the time? Do you struggle to feel satisfied after a meal?

During menopause there appears to be a connection between appetite and declining estrogen. According to *Psychology Today*, "in perimenopause, levels of the hunger-stimulating hormone ghrelin increase, a reason why many women find themselves frequently hungry during this phase. Levels of the hormone leptin, which promotes a sense of fullness, reduce throughout peri- and postmenopause." And it appears that estrogen mimics the role of leptin, so optimal levels of estrogen help keep our hunger in check. But as these levels decline, we find that we simply can't stop eating. It's like a double whammy of unfairness.

The great news is that you can retrain the way your body responds to food by focusing on specific habits that encourage you to feel true hunger before you eat and to recognize signs that indicate you are full enough. I call these hacks, and they are the focus of Chapter 7.

LOW ESTROGEN AND
THE MENOPAUSE FLESH CLOAK

At menopause we see the decline of the sex hormones estrogen and progesterone. We know that low estrogen is linked to increased belly fat, and actually that isn't such a bad thing. In fact, fat cells, also called adipose tissue, can be magnificent in the right amount. Adipose tissue is an active endocrine organ responsible for producing hormones, and it actually helps you preserve some estrogen.

Estrogen production is a complex process that I'm going to leave to the textbooks, but what you need to know is that adipose tissue does produce some estrogen and is essential in your body. Therefore, maintaining some fat during menopause is actually a good thing. There's a misconception that fat is purely used for energy storage and thermal insulation, but it does much more than that.

"Due to a loss of estrogen, fat is metabolized differently," says Colleen Keller, PhD, regents' professor and director of Arizona State University's Center for Healthy Outcomes in Aging. "It's actually laid down differently in the body as subcutaneous fat."

Menopausal women store fat more easily, especially around the abdomen, and the ability to lose it lessens. In addition to this we lose lean body mass, which is more metabolically active than fat.

Body fat can be broken down into subcutaneous fat and visceral fat. When you only put on a few pounds, they are likely to be stored as subcutaneous fat, which is the jiggly sort that you can grab that hangs over the top of your jeans and your bra strap. This shouldn't pose too many health concerns.

Unfortunately, if you gain too much weight, there's a chance it will be stored as intra-abdominal fat, or visceral fat, which is underneath your abdominal wall and can surround your vital organs. And that's a problem. We all have that uncle with the big, round, hard belly, which is usually an indicator of too much visceral fat. High belly fat is directly associated with heart disease, type 2 diabetes, and obesity, and that's why women are at higher risk for heart disease after this time. In addition, if you are overweight or obese during menopause, the chances that you will have more severe symptoms increase.

The suggested body-fat percentage for women in menopause is between 25 and 35 percent. There's a reason that one-quarter of our body is fat. Adipose tissue is crucial for our health because—as well as containing fat cells—it also contains numerous nerve cells and blood vessels, which store and release energy to fuel the body. As I mentioned, adipose tissue also releases hormones, such as estrogen, that are vital to the body's needs.

So how much fat is too much? What we're looking for is the sweet spot. Clearly, too much fat can lead to major diseases that are a blight on our health, but the right amount of fat actually helps us stay healthy, especially during menopause. If a woman's waist measures more than 35 inches, this can be an indicator for visceral fat. Visceral fat can be measured via CT or MRI scans, but these are expensive procedures.

One of the other reasons you may start to store fat in the belly area is down to your testosterone levels, which can become higher in relation to your declining estrogen and progesterone. Testosterone makes you more likely to store fat in your belly than in your hips and thighs; it's as if you start to store fat more as a male than as a female. So typically women move from a pear to an apple shape. In fact, women often see a shift in their fat distribution during menopause without ever seeing a corresponding shift in the number on the scale. Fat distribution changes throughout your life, so the fact that it moves again during menopause isn't that surprising. You are the ultimate shapeshifter.

The good news is that if you need to lose body fat, you can take action. Diet, exercise, and stress reduction (since high cortisol can increase visceral fat storage) are all proven ways to do this.

BLOATING AND WATER RETENTION

It doesn't stop there; not all your extra inches will be fat gain. Bloating and water retention are also affected by estrogen levels. As we know, the estrogen levels fluctuate throughout perimenopause, but there isn't a linear decline, so there will be times when you have higher levels of estrogen than other times. This is one of the causes of water retention, but not the only cause.

The stresses of menopause can cause problems with your gastrointestinal tract that can also be aggravated by changes in your diet, slower digestion, or other medical problems, all of which might cause you to have extra gas. Have you noticed that you are "trumpeting" a little more than usual? I am! Oh my goodness, some days I just let it rip. I get tired of trying to be discreet when all I want to do is fart continuously to relieve the pressure. I do try to restrict that to the comfort of my own home, though.

The difference between fat gain and water or gas retention is that fat is harder to lose, whereas gas and water retention are symptomatic and can be fixed. In fact, these issues usually resolve themselves as your body adjusts to its new hormonal levels. If you aren't sure which is happening, pay attention and see if you're distended throughout your tummy, holding water in your hands and feet, experiencing more gas than usual, or have worsening symptoms after eating or even at different times in your cycle. If the problem persists more than a few weeks, you should seek medical help. Some of the following suggestions may resolve bloating or water retention:

- Stay hydrated with water, but avoid fizzy drinks (except champagne, which is always acceptable).

- Avoid windy foods that might irritate or trigger these problems, such as cruciferous vegetables (broccoli, cauliflower, sprouts), some legumes (such as beans and lentils), and overly processed foods that are high in fat and salt.

- Reduce your salt consumption.

- Introduce fermented foods such as sauerkraut, kefir, and yogurt.

- Exercise regularly.

WHAT NOT TO DO ABOUT WEIGHT GAIN

As stated previously, 70 percent of menopausal women worldwide will gain weight. The knee-jerk reaction is to eat less and work out harder—that's what we did twenty years ago, so it should work now, right? Wrong. Have you ever had a vacation coming up, and realized with a panic that you had only six weeks to lose your extra weight so that you could feel good in a bikini? You probably put yourself on some kind of restrictive diet consisting of an element of starvation or physical torture: salads at most meals and tons of extra cardio at the gym. We've all been there, myself included.

The problem is that this approach doesn't work in menopause. Eating less and working out harder makes the problem worse by overloading an already stressed-out body. Remember that reduced estrogen makes us less able to cope with stress. Well, eating less and working out more are stressful to the body. What ends up happening is you find no time to rest and recover, no time to indulge in some necessary self-care. Inevitably, this leads to further weight gain. High stress absolutely sucks! In Part 2, we'll discuss strategies for managing stress, eating nutritious foods, and exercising intelligently so that you can take responsibility for your health.

WHY SOME FAT IS GOOD

Instead of looking for a body to love,
learn to love the body you are in.

UNKNOWN

I have always been worried about getting fat. I would be remiss to tell you otherwise. It is difficult growing up with media constantly telling us what healthy and fit should look like, setting unrealistic expectations for women. I was never driven by the weight on the scale, but I did experience some body dysmorphia. Although I never have looked at or will look at other women and judge them by their size or shape, it is something I've done to myself.

I think a lot of us have done this, and it is important for us to change that narrative. I have worked hard to step away from those evil thoughts in my head, and although it was a process that took time, it is achievable and very rewarding. But it always brings me back to this question: Why is it that women are so ashamed of fat, and how can we change this narrative from an evolutionary standpoint, not just a body-positive point of view?

I had a wonderful discussion on the wonders of fat with my friend Dr. Krista Scott-Dixon, from Precision Nutrition, on my podcast Fit n' Chips Chats. Talking about fat from an evolutionary point of view is very interesting; if you look back over time, fat was once considered a truly wondrous substance. Think about the paintings we see in galleries of fabulously curvaceous women lying naked on a chaise. These women were revered for their curves, but modern-day Western culture sees body fat as a problem.

As women, we perceive extra fat as evidence that our bodies have rebelled and turned against us. We are taught to despise fat and look to thin women as our inspiration and role models. Yet from an evolutionary perspective, those women signify starvation. After two million years of evolution, we have reached a place where we consider fat a problem instead of looking at the ways fat can help us. As discussed earlier, a healthy dose of fat is good for your hormonal health.

Demonizing fat and pursuing an overly lean body can be detrimental physically and mentally.

If you think your body is working against you all the time, you will never accept the natural process it is undergoing. It's not trying to mess with your head; it's trying to survive and thrive. If you change the narrative to "We are in this together as partners," understanding that evolution is simply doing its thing and that your fat storage can regulate itself with a little nudge in the right direction from you, then you can start to come to grips with some weight gain and take some unnecessary pressure off yourself.

Here are some positive things to remember about fat:

- Body fat is not just some icky, unwelcome substance that we should try to rid ourselves of; it is active and dynamic. We need some fat.

- Subcutaneous fat, located under the skin, is used for storing energy and protecting your body from hits and falls.

- Adipose tissue produces small amounts of estrogen.

Menopause is hard. It's like going through a rebirth. And this rebirth means gaining some fat. Let's learn to be in this new body as we age. Changes are going to continue to happen the older we get, and that is perfectly okay. By refusing to be frustrated and instead learning to live in your new body, you can find contentment and enjoyment.

Keep in mind why your body needs fat. Trying to stay lean is not always the healthiest option for your body. With a positive mindset it is possible to tackle the process of losing weight, if that's the right thing for you to do, to find that sweet spot that makes you *healthy* rather than *skinny*.

Okay, so you have come to grips with the fact that fat can be fabulous in the right amounts. But excessive fat can be detrimental. If you do need to lose weight, how can you do so while accepting that some weight gain is okay, but adopting good nutritional habits is still paramount? The solution to losing weight during menopause needs to incorporate four elements: nutrition, strength training, stress management, and resilience.

THERE YOU GO: all the fat facts. You've stopped hating on fat, right? We need a healthy level of fat, and science backs this up. This stage of your life finds you in a strange physiological place where your body has to do some crazy things to simply cope, adapt, and transition through menopause. Staying on top of these changes and managing the level of fat you have is very important. On the flip side, trying to lose weight if you need to is completely acceptable and is usually a requirement for maintaining good health. That's where a solid understanding of nutrition will help you, and Chapter 7 focuses on that.

PART TWO
THE HACKS

— 6 —

THE FOUR HACKS OF THRIVING IN MENOPAUSE

WHEN I SPEAK to most women about menopause, they often say that they feel overwhelmed by their symptoms but also confused by the available infor-mation about symptom relief. It is hard for them to separate the truths from the myths, to work through the contradictory information. Some of it is complete gobbledy-gook, and some of it so dry and clinical that women can't relate.

I completely get this. During my research I had to read, reread, and then read again information in books, on websites, and in scientific studies to fully understand all the medical jargon and sort through material that was chock-a-block with misinformation, bad science, and misleading statements. I just wanted to get the facts, but because menopause hasn't been taken seriously or openly discussed either in the medical field or in general conversation, it's almost as if we've all become afraid to mention it; there's an element of shame around the subject.

Today we openly discuss women's periods, but it seems that it's too embarrassing to discuss the ending of periods. How ridiculous! Thankfully, I think the tide is turning. I and other women have been talking openly about our struggles in the public realm. Radio and TV shows often have menopause discussions, and I often see menopause featured in magazines and podcasts. Finally, we are seeing progress in normalizing the conversation.

FOCUSING ON THE POSITIVE

So far this book has focused on the difficulties involved with menopause. The next four chapters focus on the positive things you can do to mitigate symptoms, to feel your best, and to be healthy.

Common things I hear women say:

"I don't need to be fixed; I just want to feel human again."

"I want to get my energy back. I'm tired of being tired."

"When will I start to feel like my old self again?"

Menopause is not something that needs fixing or curing. It's a natural process (unless it's brought on by surgery or cancer treatment) that you must go through at the end of your reproductive years and that signals a brand new phase of your life. I like to refer to it as a transformation. How you choose to go forward into that transformation is up to you. The choices and decisions you make now will determine whether you will live life to its fullest or fade into a mediocre existence.

Have you ever looked at an old photo of yourself and realized how good you really looked back then? Yet in the moment that photo was taken you only saw flaws—your wrinkles, your fat, your cellulite? We really are quite hard on ourselves in the moment, but usually in retrospect we are quite surprised at how fabulous we really were. Instead of trying to be the thirty-year-old, menopause-free self you once were, I want you to accept and love the person you are right now.

Before you start making changes in your life, it's important to acknowledge that you are a bloody amazing human being. You may not recognize the woman you see in the mirror, but that shouldn't stop you from loving everything about yourself. Being critical of yourself achieves absolutely nothing. Instead, absorb the challenge, embrace the change, and begin to enjoy life again. Accepting that you will work with where you are and who you are right now is essential to success. My plan for you is not that you will feel like your thirty-year-old self again, but that you will feel significantly better.

So what are the next steps in order to move positively forward and take control of your health?

TAKING CONTROL

If you are to fight the ravaging effects of the brain-sucking, hormone-hungry menopocalypse, you need to start taking back control of the things you *can* control. There are elements of your life that you can control, things you can do that will make the whole menopause journey easier, and to do so you need to build yourself a toolkit. Every woman will have different needs; every woman's toolkit will look slightly different. But by educating yourself on the basics of nutrition, exercise, stress management, and finding positive joy in midlife by focusing on self-care, you can finally peel off the crusty layers of menopause to stride forward majestically like the frigging cape-wearing superheroine you always knew you could be.

The journey through menopause is a process, and the things you do to help yourself thrive will change along the way. You have to go into menopause with a flexible attitude to health and wellness. As your hormones fluctuate, so must you and the things you do. It's like surfing a huge menopause wave.

Many of the symptoms discussed in the previous chapters can be relieved or controlled by making adjustments to what you eat, how you move, how you cope with stress, and how you look at your life. I have to be honest: I learned the hard way. I thought I could carry on doing everything as before and expect my body to just cope with it. I have always found it easy to rebound in my fitness and health, but menopause can put a kibosh on that.

When I get off-track, I start making tweaks here and there in my everyday life, in the areas where I have let myself go or lack focus. It may sound silly, but often for me it's about starting really small. Just refocusing on eating veggies at every meal can kick-start a whole healthy eating program. Going to the gym for ten minutes instead of my allotted forty-five starts me back on the path to building up my strength and resilience again. Although the methods I use might seem small, maybe too easy, the simple fact is: the basics work. What stops the basics from working is lack of consistency, not completely committing to the process, and quitting too soon to find the next quick fix. Integrating small adjustments into your daily life can evolve into bigger results.

I often refer to the idea of doing something consistently as "prepared readiness," setting your body up so that you are ready for anything that comes your way. Recently I decided to do a challenging four-day hike with some friends. Scaling one of the world's tallest mountains, Aconcagua in Argentina, is on my bucket list, so to help prepare myself for that, I committed to climbing the White Mountains in New Hampshire.

I currently live in Houston, Texas, and no matter how hard I look I can't see any mountains, so it was difficult for me to specifically train for this type of challenge. Instead, I just made sure that I consistently stuck to my own program. Eating well, working out enough, managing my stress so that I wasn't in a constant state of fatigue and exhaustion, and getting enough sleep—all of that made it possible for me to tackle this challenge in the best condition. I was in a state of prepared readiness that made this a fun, challenging, yet achievable adventure, and I successfully climbed the White Mountains.

We live in a world where everything is fast paced. People want the latest, fastest way to do everything, but that is the worst approach to health and wellness. None of the symptoms you are experiencing happened overnight. That extra ten pounds on your tummy didn't happen in seven days, so why would you think a seven-day cleanse was the answer to losing it?

The key is to make small but consistent changes. We tend to forget that baby steps still move us forward, and going forward is what you need to do. You are in this for the long game. Quick fixes like detox teas and skinny coffees have no foundation and are just another way the health and wellness companies prey on our insecurities.

In North America we spend more than $60 million each year on the diet industry, yet 35 percent of Americans (and 26.8 percent of Canadians) are chronically obese, costing the medical industry more than $48 billion each year. The numbers are staggering, and the personal impacts of obesity are worse—it can lead to other chronic diseases, earlier mortality, and a huge negative effect on people's quality of life. Many of these issues can be resolved by focusing on some basic things, like eating better and moving more. This cannot be achieved with false promises and expensive products. Fitness writer James Fell puts it best: "The gimmick to fat loss and better health is there is no gimmick."

Healthy lifestyle changes happen with small adjustments, or hacks. Practiced consistently, these have been scientifically proven to be the most successful way to sustain change, whether that be fat loss, stress management, or anything else you need to turn around in your life. This is how I live my life, this is how I successfully coach my clients, and it is how you will start taking control again.

Change doesn't always come easily. You cannot continue to keep doing the same things and expect change to occur. Your deeply entrenched patterns are going to be hard to break, but you can navigate around those mental obstacles by focusing on what matters to you most. And guess what? You can't make that shit just happen in a seven-day cleanse.

First, forget inspiration. Habit is more
dependable. Habit will sustain you, whether
you are inspired or not. Habit will help you finish
and polish your stories. Inspiration won't.
Habit is persistence in practice.

OCTAVIA BUTLER

THE MENOPAUSE TOOLKIT

The toolkit is made up of four hacks: how to eat, how to move, how to de-stress, and how to think. Rather than focusing on just one element of your life, I encourage you to take a big-picture, holistic view. Then, as you consistently practice the different hacks, you will see how they affect other areas of your life. For example, as you focus on improving your sleep from five hours each night to eight hours, you may find that you have renewed energy to start working out more, which in turn might motivate you to eat more intuitively. It's all connected.

Why focus on one hack at a time? Changes are easier to make when they are small and relatively easy. Focusing completely on one habit makes it easier to do it consistently, and it is the things we do consistently that actually become integrated into our lives and become automatic and habitual. If you tried to do everything in this book all at once, it would be terribly overwhelming and you would ultimately fail. If you master one change before taking the next step, the habits can build on each other. At the same time, you're keeping the number of things that require your attention each day to a minimum.

Change can be overwhelming, especially at this time of life. One of the life skills menopause has taught me is to work in manageable chunks. I no longer take on overwhelming projects that I may or may not complete and that leave me running around like a headless chicken; I have realized that I no longer thrive on that level of stress. I much prefer to take on just enough to push me to excel and not too much to stress the bejeezus out of me. It's the same with the hacks: find your Goldilocks zone.

It is inevitable that throughout our lifetime we will sometimes lose sight of what we're doing, our vision will become skewed, or our values will change. We can't always plan a perfect life, and we often have to dodge unexpected curveballs (getting sidelined with chronic symptoms of menopause, for example!). It's because of this that I encourage you to constantly re-evaluate what you need and what your body needs. At any stage in your life you can stop and revisit any of the hacks you think need more work. My point is that the story doesn't end just because the book ends. Consider this your lifetime guide into the future.

HACK 1: HOW TO EAT

Let's get completely honest here. We cannot eat the way we did in our twenties and thirties. Our bodies respond differently to food now, and therefore we have to approach eating differently. We also have to come clean and admit that what we say we're eating isn't always the same as what we're actually eating.

I am no different from you. On a Monday I can start off eating well, with full, well-rounded meals, and then by Wednesday night end up eating a bag of chips while watching the telly. So when you say you're eating really healthy food and wonder why you aren't losing weight, you need to stop and take an honest look at what you're eating.

Almost all my clients tell me they eat well but that no matter what they do, they can't lose weight. It often doesn't take too much digging to find that those little snacks in between meals (just this once), or nibbling on the kids' food as you prepare it, sipping wine while you're making dinner (just topping up the glass now and then), underestimating portion sizes (a very common problem), or enjoying that daily high-froth-crappuccino-mocha-choca-fatte-supreme can all become mindless actions that hinder your healthy eating.

Chapter 7, which is all about how to eat, reviews some nutrition basics, including what your body needs from the food you eat and how the food you eat can affect more than your waistline. In fact, fat loss is only a small part of the puzzle; eating wisely and taking time to consider your nutritional needs can also help improve your mood, your energy, your outlook on life, and your sleep. You will eat foods you enjoy. Eating should give you pleasure. It can be used to create memories or to celebrate holidays and cultural events. Removing specific foods from your diet is a method of demonizing food, which I don't endorse.

You will recall earlier in the book I spoke about how your hunger hormones are going haywire; Chapter 7 talks about understanding and relearning your body's cues. Sticking to a new way of eating can be challenging, but Chapter 7 will give you the tools to meet this challenge.

HACK 2: HOW TO MOVE

Do you do CrossFit, yoga, or Pilates? Or perhaps you run, swim, or cycle? There are so many mixed messages about which type of exercise is *the right one* to do; everybody has their opinions, and there are so many fitness fads. Remember the nineties? I was at the front of the class teaching aerobics and step, Jane Fonda–style, with my "American tan" stockings and thong leotard. And surely I wasn't the only person who owned a ThighMaster and ab roller? Oh my, those were the days!

Well, something is better than nothing. If you don't exercise at all right now, I encourage you to move in a way that makes you happy. If you find something that fills you with joy then you will likely stick to it. Recently somebody told me she had started Zumba. She was a little sheepish about admitting it to me, as I'm a huge proponent of strength training, but Zumba clearly filled her with joy. She got to dance and laugh and fill her body with those wonderful feel-good endorphins. How could I possibly hate on that?

Chapter 8, which is all about how to move, discusses what types of exercise your body needs as you age and how your body responds to it. It offers twelve weeks of strength workouts and encourages you to work with your body where it is right now and to move forward resiliently and joyfully as you age. Getting started is sometimes the hardest thing to do, but once you start you'll feel the difference between a sedentary life and a movement-filled one. Simply becoming aware of this difference can be life-changing.

HACK 3: HOW TO MANAGE STRESS

This title would have made me chuckle ten years ago. I was pretty carefree and lighthearted, so the idea of having to manage my stress would have been foreign to me. That is, of course, until I experienced the whack-a-mole hammer of menopause slamming down on me.

Managing stress can be a huge part of your life at this stage. You can be eating healthy food and exercising regularly, but if you don't find a way to manage stress, you might find yourself on a steep incline through menopause rather than cruising through the mayhem.

Stress can affect your mental health, your physical well-being, your energy levels, your ability to sleep and relax, and your ability to lose weight, among other things. During menopause, your coping skills lessen as your stress hormones go batshit crazy, so you need to take the time to make stress management an integral part of your life.

Self-care is one of the important pieces of the puzzle that are overlooked by women because they believe that looking after themselves is too time-consuming and not important enough. Yet we know that stress is a massive factor in making your symptoms worse. Taking the time to unwind, de-stress, restock (or whatever else you want to call it) is very important, and you shouldn't feel guilty about it. In Chapter 9, I give you all the tools to make this happen.

HACK 4: HOW TO THINK

Do you cringe when you hear the term self-love? It sounds so narcissistic, but that couldn't be further from the truth. The definition of self-love is simply regard for one's own well-being and happiness, a desire rather than a narcissistic characteristic. It is, in fact, self-preservation. As women, we often have many other people to take care of. How often do we put ourselves first?

Chapter 10 encourages you to put yourself first, by practicing mindfulness and identifying your values and strengths, which will build a resiliency mindset as you age. When you take care of yourself, others benefit. It's a win-win menopause scenario.

To do this, you need to learn how to become resilient in your thinking. You need to learn to age with positivity, and you need to find your own strengths and values. These are truly valuable tools that can be life-changing. Instead of focusing on society's expectations and being hard on yourself, you must learn to focus on the things you like about yourself, to change the narrative and then reach out for community support.

Before I worked with Amanda, perimenopause was a scary and almost out-of-control new phase of life. Her coaching session provided me with a valuable toolkit of skills that allow me to proactively address symptoms and actually enjoy this stage of my life.

ONLINE CLIENT

BUILDING YOUR OWN TOOLKIT

I am going to suggest you build your own menopause toolkit made up of these hacks. As we all experience menopause uniquely, your toolkit won't be the same as the next woman's, and it will change over time as your body and your health change. By using the following guide, you can scale a hack to suit your lifestyle, your needs, and your skill level.

Find your hack level: You need to find your sweet spot so that you experience a small win every time you try something new. The hack also has to be something you can implement. That may sound obvious, but jumping into new change at full throttle might make the hack hard to sustain. That's why I encourage you to find your appropriate level.

For example, say you decide to start consuming more protein, and you do so at every opportunity. By the end of week one you'll probably be sick of the sight of meat and beans. I would suggest instead introducing protein into just one of your main meals each day. So at dinner time you focus on having the appropriate amount of lean protein, and do that for two weeks until eating it at dinner time becomes second nature. Only at this stage would I then suggest increasing your protein intake at a second daily meal.

Size does matter: Start small. You are the driver, and you decide if you are ready to introduce a new hack into your life. Nobody wants to be told what to eat, when to eat it, and how much—those rigid and restrictive diet plans fail over and over again because they weren't written specifically for you!

Develop a system you can stick to: Adhering to any change is hard unless you have a system. That system can be working with a coach, finding a group of friends who keep each other accountable, giving yourself a gold star for good work, or finding an online community. There are many ways to promote success, and these are just a few examples. There's a chart below to help you track your progress; I love to give myself a tick in the box when I've achieved something I'm proud of. You should be proud of your progress and acknowledge these small steps to better health as small wins.

HACK	1	2	3	4	5	6	7	8	9	10	11	12
Hunger cues												
3 MMR workouts per week												
5 mins mind-fulness practice												

For online community support, I have a private Facebook group that I would love you to visit: www.facebook.com/groups/menopausingsohard.

The first step in making any sort of progress is to identify the tools that will help you. The second step is to know when to reach into your toolkit for help. This is usually the most challenging part. As one client told me, "Sometimes when I guess I've grown accustomed to wallowing in my depression or feelings of loneliness or whatever it is that's bothering me, I forget that I have a toolbox to reach into." Remember:

- There are always things you can do to feel better.

- Work with where you are and who you are.

- Take the judgment out of your life.

- Don't always focus on the end goal; the daily steps you take are more likely to yield results.

- Commit to a process of making improvements to your health.

- Take control of the things you can control.

OKAY, SO THERE we have the four hacks, waiting for you to get started.

By the time you finish reading this book, you will have a crap-ton of information, and you're going to know how to use it. A huge number of studies show that lasting, effective change can take you anywhere from two weeks to a year to adopt, so keep in mind that you'll be taking your time when adopting new changes. But everything you do today will affect everything you will become in the second half of your life.

By breaking things down into small steps, the changes you make will become second nature. Eventually, you will automatically know what your body needs, how to fuel and nourish it, how to care for and restore it, and how to be happy again.

— 7 —

HOW TO EAT
(HAVE YOUR CAKE
AND EAT IT!)

I N CHAPTER 5, we discussed all the reasons you might put on weight in menopause and why trying to lose weight might be more challenging than when you were younger, as well as why gaining some weight may not be such a bad thing. You may need to lose weight for optimal health, however, and this chapter will show you how to do that in a non-restrictive manner and keep excess weight off for the rest of your life.

This chapter discusses how to understand and pay attention to your body's natural cues so that you understand what it means to be hungry and when you should be feeling satisfied. This chapter also discusses the main players in the food game: protein, carbohydrates (from here on in called carbs), and fat. It also talks about your hormones and how they affect the way you process food. Then we'll pull it all together to see what that looks like in everyday life.

When I coach clients and give nutrition advice, I always start with the big no-no's. My programs have:

- no meal plans
- no restrictions
- no rigid diets
- no cheat days
- no B.S., no gimmicks
- only education you can use

The vicious cycle of yo-yo dieting comes from prescriptive, rigid thinking about food. This approach can lead to monotony, inflexibility, stress, being hangry, can lead to eating disorders, and research shows it can result in more weight gain.

GEORGIE FEAR

All we have to do is turn on the television or browse through a few books or magazines to hear about the latest keto, paleo, low-carb, grapefruit, or charcoal-chocolate diet (okay, that last one I made up) that will give you the results you want for your body. And we all have that one friend who just can't wait to tell you about their cool new diet that you just have to try. We live in a world where people love to label their diets. Wouldn't it be great if you could enjoy eating food again, guilt-free, in a way that supported your body, without the need to name it?

Some of these diets work in the short term but are unsustainable, and others are based on pseudoscience. Then you add into the mix the snake-oil peddlers selling you a diet to "fix" menopause—as if that were even possible! There is no menopause-specific diet. Your hormones cannot be reset, cleansed, or balanced, and if a diet promises to do this, then steer clear of it.

On the flip side, we have reached the point where certain food choices are vilified—gluten, dairy, fat, sugar, and carbs, to name a few. All of this can leave most people confused and unsure of what to do. This chapter provides straightforward, science-based information to help you understand the best way for you to eat. I am not going to tell you what food to pop into your mouth; I want to give you the choice. A fitness colleague of mine is fond of saying, "Telling you what to eat is like providing you the answers to a test. Sure, you'll do well on the test, but you will never learn anything."

You get to pick the foods that you want to eat, foods that you enjoy. You may have social or culturally inspired foods that you want to continue to eat. These meals are more important than just the food on the plate; they represent your culture, your heritage, and your friends and family, which likely has emotional value for you. It is possible to incorporate these foods into your diet in an intelligent way that supports your goals.

If I were to restrict the food you eat by telling you what you can or can't eat, then you would never stick to the plan. Not only are rigid diets that limit your food choices or completely omit food groups very difficult to maintain in the long term, but they can also increase your stress levels in your already stressed-out body. I have seen too many women spiral into borderline eating disorders by thinking some foods are good or bad. We are way too long in the tooth for all that crap. You need to find out which foods work best for you, which foods make you feel good. Have you ever considered thinking about food like that? How it makes you feel? The food you eat can directly affect your state of mind, your energy level or emotional capacity, and your ability to beat down menopause as you slash through symptoms like a machete-wielding Amazon warrior.

If you want to lose weight, you need to understand the principle of "calories in" versus "calories out," known as energy balance—it really is that simple. You have to consume fewer calories than you expend. But counting calories is not only time-consuming and stressful but also highly inaccurate. By learning to understand the needs of your body, you can intuitively understand what your body needs and how it responds to food. This is important if you want long-lasting results. Anybody can go balls-to-the-wall on an extreme diet for a few weeks, but after that it usually all goes to shit. Instead, together we will change the way you eat for the rest of your life.

Menopause makes losing weight challenging. Fat becomes harder to lose and seems to want to stick around longer, and we also become less efficient at using it. This doesn't mean that losing weight is impossible in menopause, it just means you need to be patient and understand how your body responds to the food you use to fuel it.

HOW TO EAT

We live in a world where we eat at such a fast pace that we barely remember what we've eaten. Watching television or being glued to our cell phones, we pay little attention to what we put into our mouths; it's of secondary importance. Long work hours mean that family meals are sometimes a thing of the past, and God forbid we might actually hold a conversation with somebody when we're having dinner. As a result of these distractions, we have stopped paying attention to the food we eat and lost the enjoyment of feeling truly nourished.

Understanding your body cues and refocusing your attention on them is a huge game-changer. Especially if you've lost sight of your health goals and don't know how to get back on track, these are very practical things you can start incorporating. And guess what? They work! But as with all new protocols, incorporating changes into your life can feel uncomfortable and be hard at first, which is why I insist that you practice the following skills for a minimum of two weeks (and chances are, you'll need more time) and try hard to stick with them. I promise you it will be worth it. You are going to learn how to feel real hunger, how to slow down when you eat, and, finally, when to stop eating.

FEEL HUNGRY

Do you eat just because it's mealtime, or do you wait until you feel hungry before you eat? Nobody wants to be hungry all the time, but a little hunger here and there can be helpful and healthy. The brain determines when you feel hungry by signaling to you that your stomach is empty and that you need to eat. Your body is an intelligent machine and wants to keep energy stores replenished. Learning to tune in to your body cues will allow you to master your hunger, enjoy your food, and eat when you actually need to eat.

Waiting until you feel true hunger, thirty minutes or so after you first feel a hunger pang, will allow you to cue into these feelings so that you know when your body is ready to be fueled. Waiting that much time will allow you to determine if what you're feeling is true hunger or if it's some other stimulus, like boredom, stress, or habit, that's making you want to eat. This puts you in the driver's seat, as you start to recognize the stimulus for true hunger.

Don't worry, you won't die! Nobody ever died from feeling hungry, though you wouldn't believe it if you met my kids. Listening to your body and letting yourself feel hunger is simply a skill you must cultivate.

If you know you've eaten and don't need any more food but are presented with a tasty snack at work, then you know it isn't true hunger that's driving you to eat it. Rather, it's a *desire* to eat. In that case, you'll have to make a choice instead of listening to your hunger cues.

Most people don't like feeling hungry. They reach for something to eat at the first sign of that grumbling tummy, or alternatively they eat just because it's mealtime, even if they're not even slightly hungry. Think about the number of times we have all eaten food without being fully engaged in the process—holidays and vacations immediately spring to mind. We eat because the occasion demands it—and I fully endorse this; why spoil your enjoyment and experience? But mindlessly eating all the time prevents the body from doing its job properly. Being hungry is a good thing to feel.

Here's how!

- When you think you're hungry, check in with yourself before you reach for food: Are you bored, anxious, or acting on an old habit?

- Let yourself feel hungry for thirty to sixty minutes before eating (more is not better).

- Start small. Practice feeling hunger before one meal a day, or practice feeling hunger for less time until you get used to it.

- Allow yourself time to get used to hunger cues. If you've been ignoring hunger and satiety cues for years, it will take time to get reacquainted with them, but they will come back.

SLOW DOWN

A report from the University of Rhode Island shows that by simply slowing down when we eat, we consume fewer calories. And we know that the only way to lose weight is to consume fewer calories than you expend.

When researchers compared the food consumption between a quickly eaten lunch and a slowly eaten lunch, here's what they found:

- When eating quickly, the women in the study consumed 646 calories in nine minutes.

- When eating slowly, the women consumed 579 calories in twenty-nine minutes.

That is sixty-seven fewer calories in twenty more minutes!

How cool is that? As simple as it seems, eating slowly really works. So slow the feck down!

In the long term, slowing down your eating is much better for your digestion than eating quickly, as it takes some of the stress away from the GI tract and allows the body to absorb the nutrients from the food, including water, vitamins, and minerals. Eating your food in a slow, controlled, and mindful manner like this allows you to enjoy the tastes and textures of your meal far more, and on top of that it helps prevent obesity. On average, twenty minutes is about enough time to signal to the brain that you've eaten enough.

Another reason it's important to take your time and know when to stop is related to your hunger hormones leptin and ghrelin, the big guns of appetite control. Sitting outside the brain, they send messages informing it when you need to eat and when you need to stop. Essentially, ghrelin is secreted in your stomach and increases your appetite, and leptin is produced in your fat cells and decreases your appetite, telling you when you're full.

Postmenopause, no matter how much fat we are carrying, our leptin levels decline, weakening the signal and leaving us feeling constantly hungry. You can counteract this by slowing down when you eat and stopping when you've had just enough.

Here's how!

- Take the time—at least twenty minutes—to eat and enjoy your food.

- Set aside time to eat.

- Take smaller bites and chew your food more.

- Put your utensils down between bites.

- Find a nice, quiet place to eat without distractions, and really enjoy your meal. Eating in front of the television or computer is distracting, preventing you from taking control of the amount of food you're consuming.

EAT UNTIL SATISFIED

When I was younger, my nanna would always leave a few pieces of food on her plate and declare out loud that she had had "sufficient." I loved the way she said this, but it was also very astute of her to recognize when to stop eating. Once you have slowed down the eating process, you will start to feel and understand the responses your body is having to the meal, rather than just chugging it all down mindlessly. Your aim should be to make sure that you feel satisfied but don't overeat, and that you digest your food well and feel better in the long run.

Learning to eat slowly, to savor the flavors and enjoy each meal, will, in my experience, help you sense when you are satisfied and avoid overeating. You know how it feels when you eat too much food: the button at your waistband starts to strain until you can't restrain the bulge any longer, you wish you had worn your stretchy pants, and you end up finishing your meal like Mr. Creosote from Monty Python's *The Meaning of Life* ("Finally, monsieur, a wafer-thin mint...") and you explode all over the restaurant. Maybe I exaggerate, but it feels rotten, and more seriously, can be detrimental to your progress.

You need to recognize what this feels like for you. Looking at the hunger satisfaction scale below, you want to learn to recognize the physical and emotional traits that put you in the Goldilocks zone in the middle column.

HUNGER SATISFACTION SCALE

STILL HUNGRY	SATISFIED	TOO FULL (MR. CREOSOTE)
Rumbling tummy	No longer hungry but not overfull	Excessive fullness
Headache/ irritability	Content to stop, even with some food left on the plate	Uncomfortable, maybe feeling sick
Potential for binge eating later	You've taken control of what you needed to eat	Feelings of regret that may lead to further overeating

Here's how!

- Stop ten to fifteen minutes into your meal and consider how you feel.

- Continue to eat slowly, chew your food, and take small bites.

- Don't feel obliged to eat all the food on your plate. If you recognize feelings of satisfaction, stop eating. One of my clients always likes to leave a few bites on her plate, which she has found a useful tool to stop her from over-indulging.

Learning to tune into your body cues takes practice, and you should not expect to be able to do this right away. You could break this down into three distinct actions: feeling hunger, eating slowly, and eating until you are satisfied. I highly recommend that you work on these three areas of eating before you start introducing dietary changes. You'll be surprised how effective this can be. This is the hack that's had the biggest impact on my clients.

WHAT TO EAT

How you eat is intrinsically linked with what you eat. My ultimate goal for you is that you learn to consume a balanced diet that provides you with satisfying meals, leaves you content and in control, and provides you with all the nutrients you need for your overall health.

Now that you have your appetite control in hand, it's time for you to make good choices based on the three macronutrients: protein, carbs, and fat. All of these need to be included in your nutrition plan, with protein and fiber (a type of carb) being the most important elements.

When you eat balanced meals, you're less likely to be struck down by cravings or to binge-eat Doritos at midnight, because your meals leave you satisfied.

(Note: many of the examples in this section come from Precision Nutrition, where I received my nutritional education—with thanks.)

PRIORITIZE PROTEIN, THE QUEEN OF FOOD

In my experience, women don't consume enough protein unless they're immersed in the fitness world. I'm not sure whether this is because of the extra work eating foods that contain protein sometimes requires—chewing a big chunk of steak can take forever—or if it's simply because of food preferences. Still, during menopause, your body is unable to use protein as effectively as before, so you need to start prioritizing protein in your daily food intake. When you do that, you will see that your hormonal shit-storm starts to calm down and you start to feel better.

Protein is the building block of life, and it's all the rage in the diet and fitness industry—we almost have an overload of information about this macronutrient. So, why is it so important to our bodies? Protein is made up of amino acids, and it's these amino acids that are responsible for producing enzymes, hormones, and antibodies. Protein helps replace worn-out cells, transports various substances throughout the body, and aids in growth and repair. Protein is also important when you're doing strength training—which builds lean muscle and increases your metabolism and which is discussed later in the book; you need protein to help you do this. During menopause and aging in general we see a larger rate of muscle loss, so consuming protein along with doing resistance training is key.

When you include more protein in your diet you will feel more satiated, and in the long term that'll make you feel happier and hopefully help you stay on course with your nutrition plan. Consuming too much protein, though, isn't necessarily a good thing—that'll only unnecessarily increase your caloric intake, so no need to go crazy. For women, I suggest a portion size that is about the size of your palm for a piece of meat or fish, or about one cup for beans or legumes, per meal. We need some protein for basic survival, and a margin above that amount to thrive, but our bodies can only store a certain amount of protein before it reaches its ceiling. Spreading your protein out throughout the day is the best way to keep your body's protein levels replenished.

As we get older, our digestive system slows down, making some proteins harder to digest. In fact, the decline of estrogen and progesterone in menopause impacts our gastrointestinal function, and our bodies become very inefficient at processing proteins. For example, the body generally finds it easier to break down fish, seafood, and eggs than steak with its tough connective tissue. Think about how you might have to chew a piece of steak compared to a piece of fish—the gastric acids in your gut face the same challenge in breaking it down. If you do enjoy eating meat and are having problems digesting it, then changing the way you cook can be helpful. Ground beef, for example, may be easier to tolerate than a dense piece of meat.

In addition to this, we know that some sources of protein, such as soy, are not as efficiently processed as others, especially in relation to building lean muscle. In her book *Roar*, Dr. Stacy Sims says, "Soy protein is not a good source of protein to increase protein synthesis and encourage lean mass development. It takes fifty grams of soy protein to match the biological effect of twenty-five grams of whey protein." Am I saying that you should avoid soy protein? Goodness no! But I do think that if you are looking to build lean muscle you will want to choose proteins that are more efficient. All protein is broken down in the body to amino acids. Whey protein contains an essential amino acid called leucine, which gets into the system fast (unlike more inefficient proteins) and can be very useful for offsetting normal age-related muscle loss.

If you're getting that afternoon slump or want some quick fuel before a workout, you will benefit from a protein-rich snack paired with a healthful carb so that you get a hit of all those wonderful nutrients and stay full for longer.

Here's how!

- Try to include good-quality protein at every meal, such as meat, poultry, fish, eggs, seafood, Greek yogurt, cottage cheese, tofu or soy foods, and whey protein or plant-based protein powders if you don't eat meat.

- For meat, fish, or chicken, use the size of your palm as your serving size at each meal. One cup of cottage cheese or Greek yogurt will also provide about the same amount of protein. Of course, you can mix and match sources, too.

- Protein is going to fill you up quickly, so avoid making this the last thing you eat on the plate. You want to make sure you eat all your protein and eat just enough other food.

- Want to stop those 2:00 PM sleepy slumps? Then make sure you consume enough protein at lunchtime and stay hydrated; you will see the difference in your energy levels.

- Consume some protein before and after exercise to ensure adequate recovery.

Here are some ideas for protein sources you can add to your meals.

Remember, as a general guideline you should aim for three to four servings per day, and one serving = the size of your palm for meats, or a cup for other sources.

- Lean meats such as beef, chicken, turkey, ground beef, pork

- Fish such as tuna, cod, scallops, shrimps, salmon

- Dairy such as eggs, cottage cheese, yogurt, cheese

- Vegan proteins including beans, peas, soy, tempeh, quinoa, nuts, seeds, and grains

- Protein powders such as whey, casein, pea, hemp, soy, and rice (to supplement your intake)

STOP HATING ON CARBS

The place to start with carbs is to understand exactly what they are. Carbs have been vilified for so long. But when you're eating a salad or a plate full of veggies, keep in mind that these are carbs too. One of the biggest issues I have with the diet culture is the message to women that "carbs are bad!" It's such a sweeping statement, with little foundation, and it's partly responsible for disordered eating.

All carbohydrates, no matter what their original source, eventually end up in your body in the form of glucose. Glucose is essential to life. The brain and central nervous system use glucose as their primary source for fuel and benefit from a continuously available supply. So you have to have carbs in your diet.

There are essentially two carb structures, simple and complex, which break further into three categories—sugar, starch, and fiber—and they all have a place in your diet. Yes, even sugar. Sugars are simple carbs and they are digested quickly, whereas fiber and starch, i.e., complex carbs, are slower to break down and are high in nutrients.

Carbs are the primary energy source for the body. They power our muscles and help us perform at our best in the gym and on the playing field. If you're an active person, cutting high-carbohydrate foods out of your diet will worsen your athletic performance, lower your energy, and compromise your immune system. Even when you're at rest, carbohydrates are the main fuel source for your brain, so they are an essential component of your diet. If you choose your carbs wisely, they will also be jam-packed full of vitamins and minerals.

Most of us equate carbs with bread and pasta, but you can also find them in dairy products (strange but true), fruits, vegetables, grains/seeds/nuts, legumes, sugary foods, and sweets. You need to choose the right carbs for maximum awesomeness.

Simple carbs

Simple carbs, or sugars (found in candy, soda, white bread, etc.), enter your bloodstream quickly, spiking your blood sugar and making you feel temporarily full. If you want to eat sugars, a good time to do it is when you're about to exercise, so that at least that sugar can help your energy levels during your workout. If you work out longer than ninety minutes, you may find that you need to consume simple carbs during your session to keep your muscles fueled.

We know that during menopause our ability to process simple carbs is lessened. Overall, too many of these carbs in our diet can make us insulin-resistant, which is not a good place to be. If you have too much sugar in your body and insulin cannot transport it to your cells for energy, then it will be converted into fat. In menopause we see increasing rates of insulin resistance, but this can be controlled to some extent by choosing complex over simple carbs most of the time. This helps control insulin response, improves body composition, and steadies overall energy level.

Simple carbs have little to no nutrient value, and they get into your system quickly. Candy, soda, white bread, crackers, and cookies are all high in carbohydrates, but they're missing the beneficial goodness of whole-food sources like oats or sweet potatoes. When we overindulge in simple carbs, our blood sugar spikes and then rapidly falls. How often have you hit that slump after a sugar rush? Additionally, a high sugar intake is associated with several chronic diseases, including obesity, diabetes, and heart disease, and it makes it harder to lose weight.

Simple carbohydrates contain either one or two molecules (hence their chemical names, monosaccharide or disaccharide), which makes them small and easy to process through the body. Some of these occur naturally in milk, but in general most simple carbs, especially in the North American diet, are added to foods. When we eat highly processed foods that have added sugar, they are likely to be devoid of any nutrient value and usually also contain added sodium and fats that do not benefit our bodies but that make the product taste really good. Overly processed foods should be significantly reduced in your diet if you want to see improvements in your weight, overall health, and energy levels.

We aren't going to completely omit the simple carbs, as these can be useful pre- and post-workout, and they're also nice treats. Everybody deserves to indulge a little. I am not telling you to cut out cakes and cookies entirely, not at all. Instead, you need strategies to include them in your diet sensibly so that you don't take all the joy out of your life! The simple rule of thumb is to eat whole foods when possible and save simple carbs for special occasions.

Here's how!

- Don't omit them completely if they give you pleasure and joy.

- Eat treats mindfully, not mindlessly; that is, plan to have them.

- When you're going to have a treat, save it for after a meal. When you're cued into your appetite control, you are less likely to overeat on treats.

- Try a smaller quantity. I am a treat snob, so I would rather have a small piece of quality chocolate than a Snickers bar.

- If it's a challenge to resist treats at home, try not buying them when you go shopping.

- Treats give us quick energy, so if you really need to eat one, do so when you need it most, like before exercising.

Complex carbs

Fiber-rich foods, such as beans, fruits, vegetables, and whole grains, contain different proportions of the two types of fiber: soluble and insoluble, and both are essential to your health. Soluble fiber keeps your blood sugar steady by slowing down the absorption of carbs into your system. It also helps to lower your blood cholesterol level. Insoluble fiber can absorb water and bulk up your stool, so essentially it promotes nice, big, juicy, soft poops. Including these foods in your diet can contribute to a healthy GI tract, and because they are so filling, they help control your appetite.

Most North Americans eat very little fiber—and that can be an ugly, uncomfortable place to be. We want to keep stuff regular, right? If you're a little bit bunged up on the loo, including grains and veggies in your diet is a very easy way to get things moving again, without having to resort to medication.

Starches are probably our most consumed type of carbohydrate and can be really beneficial in our diet. The problem is that in the modern world, many of the starches we eat are overly refined, which strips them of their nutrients and fiber content. This is where confusion seeps in. I see starches get vilified all the time, which is a pity when we know they can help with appetite suppression, that they contain fiber, vitamins and minerals, and that they can help with controlling blood glucose. I know people who actively avoid adding potatoes or rice to their meals as they deem these foods *bad*. Starches can and should have a place in your diet, as long as you pick whole-food sources. Whole-food starches are typically found in peas, corn, cereals, grains, rice, oatmeal, quinoa, and root vegetables like potatoes, yams, and butternut squash.

When we were kids, we were all told to eat our vegetables, right? In my house, we weren't allowed to eat any meat until all of our vegetables were gone, but that's a whole other story. There's a good reason we should have listened to our parents: when you include vegetables with your meals, you are loading up on nutrients including not just fiber but also phytochemicals, vitamins, and minerals. Getting those from real food beats any pill or multivitamin. And vegetables are delicious and versatile, as well as ridiculously low in calories, so eating more of them helps with fat loss because we can enjoy colorful, filling meals with very little caloric impact. No need for mini-meals when you include lots of veggies.

Including vegetables with each meal will provide you with ample amounts of vitamins A and C, which help with immune-system function and prevent you from getting every cold and flu bug that comes along. Why wouldn't you want to increase your superpowers by eating a rainbow of green, red, yellow, white, and purple veggies and helping your body fight cancer, type 2 diabetes, heart disease, and high blood pressure?

Veggies also help with your fat loss goals by increasing overall meal satisfaction. They have such high water content that they are slow to digest, meaning that you feel full while keeping your calories down. If you have a large appetite and want to continue to eat larger meals, load up on your vegetables.

So be sure to eat plenty of complex carbs. Your insides will thank you for all that additional soluble and insoluble fiber you are providing, especially as fiber may help with lowering cholesterol and preventing colon cancer as well. And the benefits of all those vitamins and minerals are almost too plentiful to count. Bet you can't wait to eat some broccoli now (unless it makes you fart; seriously, gut issues in perimenopause are no joke!).

Here's how!

- The best way to get complex carbohydrates into your meals is to include plenty of vegetables. At each meal make sure you have a variety of veggies, with a good size portion being the size of your fist, but feel free to add more if you're especially hungry. I often have a ginormous salad, where half my plate is filled with veggies.

- Don't forget a starch. Include a smaller amount of whole grains, peas, corn, or potatoes with your meals. A good portion size is a cupped hand at each meal. For example, have oatmeal with breakfast (I call it porridge but this isn't the time to argue), bread with lunch, and rice with dinner.

- When you're less active your body needs fewer carbohydrates and calories, and when you're more active your body needs more. You might find it works best for you to have your highest-carbohydrate meals either just before or just after your workouts to ensure strong performance and rapid recovery.

- Try to choose unprocessed or minimally processed foods as much as you can. Each step in processing can mean added sugars, preservatives, flavors, and colors, and loss of fiber and nutrients. Additionally, you save money by choosing bananas or rice for your carbs instead of overpriced granola bars.

Here are some ideas for complex carb sources you can add to your meals.

For complex carbs, your serving size is at least one or two fistfuls for veggies or a cupped handful for other sources, at each meal.

- All kinds of colorful veggies, including broccoli, green beans, leafy greens, celery, peppers, cucumbers, and carrots

- Bread, grains, rice, pasta, oats—where possible choose minimally processed, whole-grain varieties

- Potatoes, sweet potatoes, corn, beans, lentils, peas

- Fruit, all varieties

EAT FAT

Yeah! I said it: Eat fat! Eating fat will not make you fat. Taking in too many calories is what makes us gain weight.

There are so many misconceptions about fat: Do you remember the advice on low-fat diets from the eighties and nineties? Even today people are still scared to eat and enjoy fats as they should. Fats play an important role in our bodies, and we should mindfully include them in our daily meals. Conversely, overconsumption of any fats, but in particular saturated fats, may lead to obesity and other health problems. Therefore, determining the optimal amount is important.

The main reason we should eat fat is that it tastes so damn good! (Mmm, butter!)

Besides that, though, we get many health benefits from consuming fats, and they play a vital role in keeping us healthy. They are required for metabolism, absorption of nutrients, and cardiovascular health; they help to satisfy hunger; and certain fats have been shown to help alleviate depression.

Some fats are not optimal for your health, however; trans-fatty acids (AKA trans fats) should be avoided completely. There are two types of trans fats. Natural trans fats are produced in the guts of some animals, and some foods produced from them may contain small traces of naturally occurring trans fats. These are fine to consume. Artificial trans fats (trans-fatty acids) are industrially manufactured by adding hydrogen to vegetable oils to turn them into solids. They are cheap to produce, have an endless shelf-life, and are tasty, so the public keeps wanting more of them.

Unfortunately artificially produced trans fats have been shown to increase your LDL (*bad*) and lower your HDL (*good*) cholesterol levels, which puts you at an increased risk of heart attack, stroke, and diabetes. The good news is that both the FDA and the WHO have made moves to ban trans fats. They are currently banned in America and some other countries around the world. In November 2015, the FDA determined that partially hydrogenated oil is no longer Generally Recognized As Safe (GRAS) and gave manufacturers until 2018 to eliminate it, though some companies have extended that time by a few years. Because of these exemptions, some foods might still contain trans fats, like shortening, margarines, frozen pizzas, pie crusts, cookies, and fast foods, but soon they will be completely eliminated. My advice: do not eat them, ever!

Fats fall into three categories: saturated (found in butter and animal fats), polyunsaturated (seeds and fish), and monounsaturated (nuts and avocado), and a variety of each should be included in your daily meals. By adding fats to your fruits, vegetables, carbohydrates, and lean proteins, you should be able to reach this goal. It is important not to have too much saturated fat, and certainly not to have only saturated fat, in your diet. Make sure you enjoy a smorgasbord of fats.

The bottom line: enjoy fat, eat a variety of fats, and get it from real food sources. It will help you feel fuller after your meals and make the food taste really good!

Here's how!

- Include fats from whole, high-quality foods in all of your meals, and be sure to include a variety of fats.

- If you are struggling to meet your daily fat allowance, consider adding some olive oil or peanut butter, for example, to your diet.

- Most people could benefit from additional omega-3 fatty acids, which are mainly found in fish. If you aren't eating fish a couple of times a week, consider taking a good-quality fish oil each day.

Here are some ideas for fat sources you can add to your meals.

As for serving size, let's keep it simple. It's difficult to measure fat servings as most of it is contained within the food you are eating or added as part of the cooking process. An easier way of including fats in your diet is to eat a variety of different food sources. Here are some examples:

- Animal fat from eggs, meat, butter, cheese, fish
- Nuts, seeds, avocado, olives
- Fish oil, flax oil, coconut oil, olive oil, and other cooking oils

Remember that many foods already contain fats, so you may not need to add extra fat to your meal. Too much added fat will just mean too many extra calories.

DRINK WATER AND LIMIT YOUR BOOZE

Let's start with water—the elixir of life. I am a water fanatic. I encourage everybody to increase their water consumption, because so many people are dehydrated and don't know it. If it's two o'clock in the afternoon and you start to feel really sleepy, you might assume you need more sleep or caffeine. There's a good chance, however, that you are dehydrated. When you're dehydrated, your cognitive performance suffers dramatically. Dehydration by as little as 1 percent of your body weight (two pounds for a two-hundred-pound person) is enough to reduce both endurance and strength.

Your body is made up of 60 percent water. Water is essential for a variety of physiological functions, including transporting nutrients and maintaining proper body temperature, as well as bowel function. Your overall health, performance, and body composition will suffer if you don't adequately hydrate. So let's start glugging!

You may also instinctively reach for food when in fact your body is just dehydrated. Conversely, if you are hungry, drinking water will usually take the edge off that hunger. If you aren't sure whether you need food or water, drink some water first and see how you feel in fifteen minutes. The water won't hurt, and maybe you don't need to eat just yet anyway. In some studies, participants who drank water before they ate their meals lost three to five pounds over a twelve-week period.

I'm a water purist, but that doesn't mean you have to be. In fact, drinking tea, coffee, and flavored water is also okay; just be sure to pay attention to the sugar content of these drinks. It seems silly to drink away your calories if you don't need to. In addition, if you've increased your fruit and veggie consumption, you'll be happy to know that they are full of water—so be sure to keep including them in your meals.

This is usually a hard hack for people to get used to, so start slowly. Take water with you wherever you go for the first week or two. When you have your cup of water nearby, you're more likely to sip away.

Your body has a neat way of keeping you informed if you have drunk enough fluid: if you aren't thirsty or if your urine is colorless/pale, you are likely hydrated enough.

Now, on to booze. You may notice that as you get older, you become more intolerant to the effects of alcohol on your body. I can't drink very much these days, and I am ok with it. Sure, I would like to feel a bit squiffy occasionally, but dealing with a terrible hangover (and for me a migraine) after just one or two drinks really isn't worth it. And I know many of you agree. Many women in my online community say they've also noticed that their tolerance for booze has decreased. This might be down to age or menopause or both, but your body will thank you for moderating your consumption.

There are many health reasons for doing this, and reducing your intake might also help alleviate some of your menopause symptoms. NAMS reports that excessive drinking can lead to increased risk of some cancers; increased menopause symptoms like hot flashes, anxiety, depression, and insomnia; weight gain, which can lead to a risk of heart disease; and an increased risk of osteoporosis. Alcohol may also interact adversely with medications you are taking.

So what does excessive drinking mean? The National Institute on Alcohol Abuse and Alcoholism (NIAAA) defines one standard drink as

- 5 fluid ounces (one glass) of wine (about 12 percent alcohol). Don't let your wine glass fool you—most hold much more than 5 ounces.

- 12 fluid ounces (usually one can or bottle) of regular beer (about 5 percent alcohol)

- 1.5 fluid ounces (one shot) of 80-proof distilled spirits

For women, it defines moderate (low risk) drinking as no more than seven drinks per week and no more than three drinks on any single day. If you exceed this amount, you are considered a heavy drinker and are open to the associated health risks.

Moderation is key, and that might mean drinking a lot less than you thought.

Here's how!

- Ideally, aim for half your body weight in ounces of water per day. For example, a woman weighing 140 pounds should drink 70 ounces, or approximately 2 liters, of water each day.

- On days when you exercise, consider adding another 25 to 35 ounces to that amount.

- Try drinking water before and during your meals to help curb your appetite.

- If you start feeling sleepy, try drinking water to see if you become more alert.

- If you're not used to drinking water frequently, sometimes investing in a fancy-pants drink container can encourage you to drink more.

- Restrict your alcohol consumption to no more than seven drinks per week and no more than three drinks on any single day—and even less if you want to lessen your health risks and menopause symptoms.

PUTTING ALL THAT TOGETHER

How you eat and what you eat matters. Eating according to the guidelines set out in this chapter will improve your relationship with food and put you in the driver's seat to make better choices and stay in control. Your relationship with food is important and should be a positive experience; yet we know that most diets thrive on instilling fear and creating a negative attitude toward food. I encourage you to add food that nourishes you to your diet rather than looking for items you can remove—for example, look for ways to add more protein to each meal rather than removing carbs.

Losing weight in menopause can be a struggle, and most women give up before they learn how to moderate their consumption by using cues to understand when they're hungry and when they're satisfied. This takes a lot of patience, especially when you don't see immediate results. How many times have you said to yourself, "I'll start again after the weekend?" I know I have. Well, how about changing that narrative, and just starting now? Even if you aren't successful all of the time, just keep forging ahead. I promise you, this will work for you.

Let's review what you've learned in this chapter. Remember to pick an action that you think you can be successful at, stick with it, and track it to hold yourself accountable.

HOW TO EAT

- Eat when you're hungry.

- Eat slowly; take around twenty minutes to finish a meal.

- Eat until you're satisfied.

WHAT TO EAT

- Keep your protein intake consistent, consuming some protein at all meals.

- Load up on your veggies; use these to fill up your plate.

- Make sure to include a variety of other complex carbs (grains, peas, corn, rice, pasta, etc.) and fats in your meals.

- Limit simple carbs to around the time you exercise and for treats.

- Stay hydrated.

- Limit alcohol consumption.

— 8 —

HOW TO MOVE (THE MMR WORKOUTS)

ONE OF THE reasons I'm such an avid supporter, as I've mentioned, of strength training for women is because of the impact it has had on me. Becoming strong has transferred over to my everyday life. There is no downside. Being able to lift weights heavier than my own body weight is so empowering that it has improved my confidence outside the gym. It has also improved my energy level, my mental health, and my overall body image. Instead of paying so much attention to the number on the scale, I am now focused on the amount of weight I can lift.

Too often, we think of strength building as something for vanity-seeking glamor girls and bro-science meatheads in the gym. That's a pity, because it has such a positive effect, no matter who you are. I've seen my female clients become more confident and courageous outside of our training sessions. They try new things or take on new challenges, both at work and at play, and overcome obstacles they never thought they could.

From the age of thirty onward, you start to lose muscle mass at the rate of around 2 to 3 percent each year. This is called sarcopenia. The main cause of sarcopenia is from leading a sedentary life, but when menopause comes into play, you will find your declining hormones can also accelerate your loss of muscle mass, which affects your power, strength, balance, and aerobic capacity.

That sounds bad, right? Well, yes, it isn't great, but all is not lost. It is important to understand how losing muscle can affect you and your health and why it's important during menopause for you to strength-train and build muscle.

There seems to be a general misconception that older women can't get strong, that we can't build muscle after menopause. This couldn't be further from the truth. It is possible; menopause just makes it harder. During menopause, muscle protein synthesis—your ability to build muscle—is lessened, which requires you to focus more on the type of exercise you choose and the way you feed your body to support growth (remember all my talk about protein in the last chapter?).

Women often get scared at the thought of lifting weights, not only because they fear they might get bulky (they won't), but also because it looks so intimidating. By the end of this chapter I hope you'll feel joy instead of fear about your workouts and will look forward to working out and feeling empowered.

Exercise should bring you happiness, not make you miserable. I hope you will find the exercises in this chapter fun (just wait until you read my exercise cues). Society has fed us the narrative that women need to remain as small and thin as possible. Conversely, lifting weights encourages us to take up a lot of space—and that's a good thing. Lifting weights makes you realize that you're capable of more than you ever imagined. You will see measurable achievements as you progress, and that will calm all of those negative thoughts.

THE IMPORTANCE OF STRENGTH TRAINING DURING MENOPAUSE

It's complicated. The idea of growing old—of becoming fragile and not being able to move well, lift objects, or function as an able-bodied person—horrifies me. Strength training allows you to perform such tasks easily and without fear of injury. Of course, there are the aesthetic benefits, too—we all want to look good—but the primary reason to strength-train is that your body needs it.

One of the first things your body starts to lose as you age is your power output, followed closely by your strength. Power is both strength and speed together. Picture yourself as a hundred-meter sprinter; you must not only be fast but also have the strength to carry yourself to the finish line. Okay, I hear you; you have no intention of sprinting a hundred meters. So why do you need to focus on improving your power and strength?

During menopause, you have an increased risk of a number of diseases and physical problems, including osteoporosis, diabetes, high blood pressure, joint pain, and injury. Strength training plays a huge role in keeping those conditions at bay.

Falls are one of the main reasons the elderly visit the emergency room, and falls are caused by poor balance and lack of strength. I don't want to be another statistic as I grow old, and neither should you.

Strength training makes everyday tasks easier to do. Power training helps you move quickly and react to falls. Both help you feel capable and empowered.

(And strength training really helps you have a good butt.)

Remember that it's more important than ever to pay attention to your protein intake and try to include protein at every meal. This, along with strength training, can help offset the loss of strength and power.

I've mentioned before that you can have higher relative levels of testosterone in your body during menopause, and we usually associate testosterone with people like Arnold Schwarzenegger, who have muscles on top of their muscles. So if we have more relative testosterone, isn't it easier for us to build muscle in menopause? Unfortunately, the answer is no. Your ability to build up and break down protein is totally out of whack, so it's not doing its job as efficiently as before. We need that protein to build muscle, so all of a sudden the process becomes much harder than when you were premenopausal. The good news is that you can still build muscle, but now you need a little more patience and dedication and a great nutrition and workout program (I've got you covered).

MISCONCEPTIONS ABOUT STRENGTH TRAINING

BUILDING LEAN MUSCLE HELPS YOU LOSE WEIGHT

This is true(ish). Building lean muscle will indeed help boost your metabolism, but it's not the answer for losing weight. To lose weight you need to pay attention to your food intake—that must always be your priority. Abs are made in the kitchen! But it's true that muscle is metabolically active, so it uses the food you put into your body as fuel more efficiently. Combining good nutrition with building lean muscle is a win-win for weight loss.

WOMEN WILL GET BULKY LIFTING WEIGHTS

Codswallop! If you still think you'll get big from lifting weights, I want you to go over to a wall and bang your head against it to rid yourself of that idea. Because your body's dynamic makeup, or physiology, is so different from a male's, it's just not possible—without the aid of chemically enhanced substances—to get bulky. In fact, the inverse is likely to happen. Because muscle is more compact and shapely than fat, you are probably going to get smaller. Building lean muscle is a wonderful way to create a great body shape and a more finely tuned engine.

A POUND OF MUSCLE WEIGHS LESS THAN A POUND OF FAT

Seriously, I hear this all the time! Read it again. How can a pound weigh less than a pound? Questions like this make my head hurt. A pound of muscle clearly weighs the same as a pound of fat. I believe what people are thinking when they say this is that a pound of muscle is significantly *smaller* than a pound of fat. Muscle is compact and generally takes up less space. That's why women who start strength training often see their dress size shrink even though the numbers on the scale remain the same.

THIS IS A good time for me to remind you that you should focus less on the weight on your scale and more on the weight of the dumbbell you use. Women are hyper-obsessed with having a smaller, lighter body and put too much focus on the scale. Strength training shifts that focus to a more significant measurement—how much weight you can lift!

Once you've started strength training, your new metabolically active body will have improved insulin sensitivity—meaning that the cells of your body will use blood glucose more effectively—and cardiovascular output, as well as a better ability to fight heart disease, some cancers, and osteoporosis. We know about the last because physical activity, particularly weight-bearing exercise, provides the mechanical stimulus, or "loading," that is important for the maintenance and improvement of bone health and muscle loss.

Osteoporosis (brittle bones) and osteopenia (less severe bone loss) are major health risks for postmenopausal women—the stats are frightening. Just being a woman puts you at a higher risk of having osteoporosis. In the United States, one in two women over fifty (i.e., postmenopausal) are likely to break a bone, according to the National Osteoporosis Foundation. A woman's risk of breaking a hip is equal to her combined risk of breast, uterine, and ovarian cancer, and 21 percent of elderly people who break a hip will die within a year as a result of complications. That statistic is really scary. Strength training provides you with the stimulus to both build and maintain bone strength and protect your skeleton with increased lean muscle.

Sarcopenia, as I mentioned, is muscle loss that occurs with aging and being sedentary—our muscle mass degrades by 2 to 3 percent annually after the age of thirty. Losing muscle affects our basic functions like walking, balance, and the ability to get up after we fall, and our flat-lining hormones play a role in muscle loss, too. So can we slow the aging process? Good news, my friend: yes, we can. With a focused strength program and great nutrition protocols, you have this problem covered and you can start today.

Another benefit of strength training is that it can help improve your posture, and that in turn will help prevent injury—which we see so much of in our midlife onward.

Biochemically, when your body becomes stressed it's more likely that you'll get injured. The opposite is true when you improve your lean body mass: when your body is stressed, you rebound more quickly. The muscles you build protect your body; when you push your muscles through discomfort, and a little harder than before (both of these in a positive way), then you recover better if you already have a base of lean muscle.

Lastly, two fabulous studies have been published that show how strength training and having lean muscle can help vasomotor symptoms in menopause. While working out at the gym, Dr. Rosanne Woods noticed that her friends who were the quintessential "cardio-bunnies" were the women who were complaining about their severe menopause symptoms, most specifically hot flashes and night sweats. So she decided to conduct research to look at the association of lean body mass with menopausal symptoms. The study found that maintaining a higher lean body mass (defined as your body weight minus your body fat) is the greatest contributing factor to reducing menopause symptoms. The study recommends that all women do strength training regularly for as long as possible, and it encourages us to start early as a preventive measure.

The second study looked at postmenopausal women, with no HT, who started pumping iron, and it found that their hot flashes decreased. Fifty-eight women who averaged 7.5 hot flashes or night sweats per day took part in a fifteen-week resistance program. They were challenged to work harder than they'd typically worked out before, and the results showed that their symptoms reduced by 50 percent to an average 4.4 episodes a day. Studies like this can be very helpful to women who cannot take HT—for example, breast cancer patients, who really struggle with vasomotor symptoms. This shows that strength training is an actionable step they can take to help improve how they feel.

Sometimes a strength training program can bring transformations beyond the physical, and this saved my sanity during menopause. I have spoken openly about my struggles with depression, and strength training proved to be one of the best ways to help boost my mood and give me back some of my mojo. When you strength-train, your body produces two anti-depression biochemicals, serotonin and endorphins, which have been shown to have a positive effect on some forms of mental illness, including depression. For me, it was part of my survival plan. Talk about empowerment!

I recently spoke with Dr. Susan Kleiner, a sports nutritionist, and she pointed out that with middle age comes fear or an unwillingness to step out of your comfort zone. "When it comes to moving well, when the belief that you can do things again has left you, it will translate to loss of lean body mass," she says. "It's important to remember that it's in the challenge where the magic happens, where we make progress. Advantage comes in the challenge rather than doing just what you can do. So if you're not moving forward, then you are just moving backward. A huge part of this is the training: the willingness to be uncomfortable to face or overcome fears and real athletic challenges. Also, what happens biochemically is that when we stress the body, it rebounds stronger. Physiology: that is how we recover."

Exercising shouldn't be a chore. It should be something that you want to do, that you enjoy doing. This program will cover those bases. I've learned that finding time to make myself a priority in life not only makes me physically feel better but also results in improved cognitive behaviors, improved sanity, and a sense of empowerment. Remember, if you build a strong body you are protecting your joints, and you're building a system of muscles that can contract, react, and bounce back, helping you stay injury-free and mobile, as well as fighting diseases such as osteoporosis, diabetes, and heart disease.

DON'T LET THE OLD LADY IN

There's a popular song by Toby Keith called "Don't Let the Old Man In." I was recently speaking to a friend at the gym who is seventy-three years old and is a shining example of what a healthy person can achieve as they age. He works out four times a week, with a positive energy that impacts everybody around him. I asked him his secret, and he told me that when he gets down, is tired, or lacks motivation, he tells himself, "Don't Let the Old Man In."

I had to remind myself of this recently. After three months of poor health and diminished mojo following a bout of chronic migraines, I really started to think I'd never feel fit and strong again. I felt exhausted and humbled by my inability to work out, eat well, or feel enthusiastic about anything, but I also knew that this wasn't how it was supposed to be. These migraines came out of the blue and sidelined me. I was eventually referred to a neurologist and he established that the problem was down to my hormones! Jesus, they really just do keep on giving. I adjusted my HT dose with my gynecologist, started some migraine medication, and eventually felt human again.

One of the few things that got me through was a gentle reminder to myself that I had to be more than how I was feeling and that I knew I could be fighting strong again.

Once I was back to feeling well again, building up my strength and enjoying my workouts, I started constantly telling myself, "Don't Let the Old Lady In."

This is just one of the lessons menopause has taught me. It's a tough ride, but it's one that brings clarity to my health goals. I plan to age positively with resiliency and strength. You can, too.

THE IMPORTANCE OF NEAT

In addition to introducing strength workouts into your life, I'm also going to encourage you to actively recover. Menopause has us walking that fine line of stress, with cortisol always present in the background. By keeping our workouts short, hard, and fast (coincidentally, that's exactly how I like my men!) you will not elicit a huge cortisol spike and therefore won't be utterly exhausted afterward—but you still need to prioritize your recovery. We talk more about stress in the next chapter, but for now I just want to acknowledge that recovery after exercise is important to a more sane existence in menopause. NEAT is part of that recovery.

NEAT stands for non-exercise activity thermogenesis. Simply put, it means all the movement you do that isn't exercise.

Each day your body has to use calories for different things; your calorie needs aren't just for exercise. The total number of calories your body needs each day is called total daily energy expenditure (TDEE), and it's made up of several elements: TDEE = BMR + TEF + NEAT + EAT

- *BMR, or basal metabolic rate.* This is the calories it takes for you just to exist. It accounts for up to 60 percent of the total calories you use, even if you just lie in bed all day and never do anything else, absolutely no activity. Isn't that crazy?

- *TEF, or thermic effect of food.* It takes calories for the body to consume calories. Remember the story about how eating celery burns more calories than the celery itself contains? Not sure how much truth there is in that, but still your body uses around 10 to 15 percent of your total calories to digest the food you eat.

- *NEAT, or non-exercise activity thermogenesis.* This is all of the everyday movement that isn't part of your workouts. We will dig a bit deeper into this now.

- *EAT, or exercise activity thermogenesis.* Your workouts! You really can't rely heavily on this portion of the day to "torch your calories." Of course exercising does use up energy, but you may be surprised to see this is the smallest part of your overall expenditure.

NEAT can account for as little as 15 percent of your total calories burned if you are very sedentary (and we all have those days) but up to 50 percent in very active individuals. Can you see where I'm going here?

NEAT activities could be things like cleaning, shopping, walking, or running around like a headless chicken when you have too much to do.

Let's run some numbers. I'm going to use simple numbers for ease of math, just so you get the concept.

If a woman has a TDEE of around 2,000 calories, her BMR will be approximately 1,200, and she'll burn about 200 calories to digest the food she eats each day (TEF). And her NEAT will range from 300 to 600 calories more per day depending on whether she spends the day sitting and working on the computer or if she has a day full of walking, shopping, and generally moving

So without any intentional exercise, she would burn around 1,700 calories if her NEAT activities are on the low end, and 2,000 on the higher end.

That's a 300-calorie-per-day difference between her sitting at the computer or going for a couple of walks. Moving every day helps you burn calories and it's why you see people panicking to get their 10,000 steps in.

Consider this: the average calories burned during an hour of intentional exercise is about 325 calories for every hundred pounds of body weight (so a 150-pound woman burns about 490 calories by working out hard for an hour). Now, most of us aren't engaging in a solid hour of nonstop exercise every day. If that 150-pound woman does thirty minutes on the elliptical, she's only burning, on average, 245 calories. That's about the amount in two tablespoons plus a smidge of almond butter (which isn't that much!). But get this: if she adds an active walk for an hour, she can burn an additional average of 300 calories.

This is not an invitation not to exercise and just go shopping all day. There are many benefits to working out. We know it helps promote HGH (human growth hormone), raise endorphins, reduce stress, build lean muscle, and boost metabolism, to name but a few. Yet we can see that the activity outside of our workouts is very important too.

What does this mean for you?

It means you need to move. Sitting around all day is killing us. I highly recommend that you focus some time on your NEAT. So if you're having a non-workout day because you don't feel up to it, or it's a rest day in your schedule, I encourage you to move in a way that's fun and that gets your blood pumping and your endorphins flowing. Walking is a beautiful way to do this: actively walking outside in nature for an hour can help you burn some extra calories, boost your mood with feel-good hormones, and be with nature—which is always a good thing to do, as it lowers the stress that riddles our body during menopause.

Make NEAT a serious priority in your life. You need it.

A NEW WAY TO WORK OUT

I have talked a lot about the importance of strength training as we age. This is not just about looking good naked (or in your clothes); it's about conditioning your body with enough load and aerobic challenge to ensure that you support your joints, limit the possibility of injury, help prevent chronic disease, and be strong, which then translates into your everyday existence and keeps you young. (The pert bottom doesn't hurt, either.)

When you work out you need to challenge your muscles, to create changes in their structure that will result in improved stability throughout the body, improved metabolism, and improved health. I am excited to introduce you to my workout series, called Menopause Metabolic Resistance (MMR).

Every single MMR workout will improve your strength, power (strength and speed), and cardio output for a healthy heart—all important things that must be made a priority as we age. This means you'll be training with weights that are heavy enough to create a stimulus, which helps improve coordination, and fast enough to get you out of breath. There's a ton of research to back up these workouts, and I've taught these techniques to hundreds of clients. All of these workouts last between twenty and thirty minutes. I recommend that you try to schedule at least three workouts from the series each week.

I encourage you to push yourself to lift more weight than you previously thought you could. Know and trust that you can push a little harder. I suggest that you start with light to moderate weights—at least until you get comfortable with the new exercises and you nail your form. But to create the changes you need to see, you have to be willing to push to a higher limit.

Here's how that looks: if you're doing a rep range of ten exercises, by rep eight you should start to be fatigued, and by rep ten you should barely be able to push out that last rep. When you start to understand this level of fatigue, you will start to see the benefits usually within a few sessions—you'll be amazed at the results, I promise you. If you own a pair of little pink ankle weights, well, the nineties called; they want them back!

Okay, let's get to the workouts! I bet you can't wait.

This chapter includes:

1. Quick and effective workouts that last between twenty to thirty minutes

2. A workout schedule to help you adhere to the program of three times each week—yes, that's enough!

3. Three phases of workouts that will last a minimum of twelve weeks all together

4. Easy-to-perform exercises that use multiple muscle groups, sometimes called compound exercises, which make you more efficient with time and the number of reps you need to perform

5. Multiple planes of motion and resisting of forces, getting you moving in lots of different directions with differing speeds and resistance—you know, just like in real life

6. Exercises that promote both strength and power, two things that diminish as we age

7. Joint-friendly exercises that don't put excessive strain on your lower back, knees, or shoulders

8. Single-legged exercises to improve balance and stability

9. Core work that will help build a solid base in the front, back, and sides of your trunk, to protect your spine and help your shoulders and hips move better

10. Fun! (These are fun. You'd have to be dead inside not to enjoy these workouts.)

HOW TO MAKE IT WORK FOR YOU

- Create a schedule that you can adhere to and be honest with yourself. I am asking you for three sessions a week for thirty minutes maximum. If George Clooney asked you to clear your diary for a two-hour lunch, you would do it. Do this for you!

- Make it personal by performing the number of rounds based on where you are with your fitness and energy levels:

  › Beginner: Three circuits per workout

  › Intermediate: Four circuits per workout

  › Advanced: Five circuits per workout

- Buddy up if it helps you stick with the plan. Working out with friends is always more fun and is usually a great way to stay motivated.

- Play around with my suggested schedule at the end of the chapter. If working out on back-to-back days is more convenient and suits your energy levels, then do it. If alternating days is more your style, then that works too.

- This workout plan is perfect for the absolute beginner or for somebody who has taken some time away from fitness. It's also great for the seasoned athlete. Even though the exercises are relatively simple, they are all effective. This is how I work out. Within the program I give you ideas for how to pimp it up if you want to push a little harder.

WHAT YOU WILL NEED

- Two pairs of dumbbells or kettlebells (as Arnie says, your muscles don't know what you're holding, so feel free to work out with your medium-sized dog... #joke). One pair should be moderate weight that you can lift overhead for 8 to 10 reps—in the ten-to-fifteen-pound range. The second pair will be a heavier weight that you can squat 8 to 10 reps with—in the twenty-to-thirty-pound range.

- A yoga mat.

- A bench or chair (required for certain exercises; check your workout plan for the day).

- Water.

- Funky music to get you pumped up for action.

- Workout clothes. You don't need to run out to Lululemon just yet, but please make sure you're wearing something comfortable that allows you full range of movement.

- Flat-soled trainers or bare feet (this is my preference) so that you can feel the floor below you.

- Attitude. Treat these workouts seriously. Create an environment that makes you want to exercise.

Now let's go!

FORM MATTERS!

Before you head into the workouts, focus on these training tips, which will help you get the most out of your workouts.

Dynamic warm-up: Spend five minutes at the start of each workout preparing your body.

Engage your core: When I tell you to engage your core, imagine I'm going to sucker-punch you in the gut, and you tense up to try to stop it from hurting. That's how you engage your core. You don't have to be as dramatic as that, but understand what that sensation feels like.

Squeeze your butt: Stand up straight and imagine you have a $100 bill between your butt cheeks. I am going to try to remove it, so squeeze your cheeks together to stop me. That's what I want you to remember when I tell you to squeeze your butt.

Activate your feet or hands: Movement starts from the ground up. So if your hands or feet are touching the ground, I don't want them to be passive. I want you to imagine that you're trying to pick up the floor, so that your knuckles or toes turn white and you see the tendons stand out. When you create activation, you prepare the rest of your body for movement.

Squat versus hinge: It's not uncommon to get these two movements mixed up, and you see both of them a lot in my workouts. They're both fundamental movements that we load up with weights in the workouts. A hinge is where you break at the hips and send your butt backward, usually with a slight bend in the knee. A squat is where you bend your knees and take your hips toward the floor, much like squatting on a potty.

How much weight to use: Each workout lists the number of reps you should do of each exercise. If I ask you to do 8 to 10 Goblet Squats, then the dumbbell you use should be heavy enough that by rep 8 you're working hard, with the last two reps seeing you push hard to the end. If you can comfortably do 12 to 15 reps with that weight, then you need a heavier weight.

When to rest: All of the exercises are performed in a circuit. Don't take a break between exercises; wait until the end of each complete circuit and then rest one to two minutes before starting again.

DYNAMIC WARM-UP

This dynamic mobility sequence is the perfect way to prepare your body for your MMR workout. It's a set of four exercises that you link together in a flow. The purpose of the flow is to warm up the body and prepare your joints without using static stretches. You simply move from one exercise to the next, after performing the prescribed number of reps, without stopping. You can also use the dynamic warm-up on your days off; it's a great way to get the joints oiled and the blood flowing.

Overhead Squat

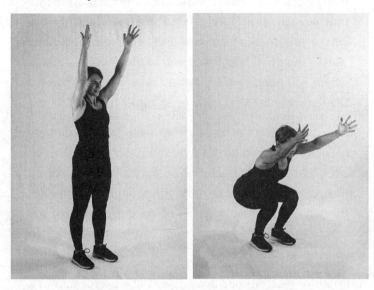

With your arms overhead, without shrugging your shoulders, squat down as far as you can. Don't worry if the body tips forward, this is perfectly normal, but try to keep as relaxed as possible in this position. Stand straight back up, keeping your arms overhead the whole time. *Do this 5 times before moving onto the next exercise.*

Inchworm

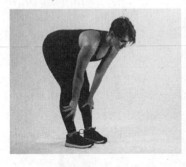
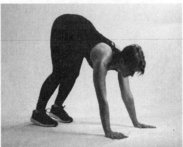

From standing, place your hands on your shins and bend your knees as much as you need to to reach the floor. Now start walking your hands out until your body reaches a full plank position. Then reverse the action until you're back to full standing. On the last rep, remain in a plank position. *Do this 5 times before moving onto the next exercise.*

Plank to Crouch

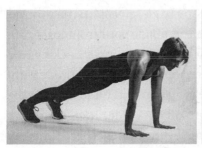
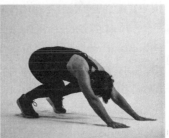

From a plank position, bend your knees and push back with your hands so that your body moves backward into a crouch position. You should be high on your toes and sitting back on your haunches. Don't worry about how deep you get into this exercise; you're simply creating movement through the ankle, knee, and hip joints. Come back to plank position. *Do this 5 times before moving onto the next exercise.*

Half-Kneeling T-Spine Reach

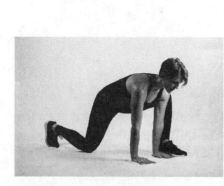 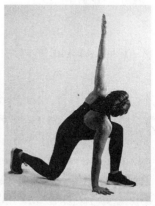

From a plank position, bring your left foot forward beside your left hand, and drop your right knee down—this looks like a runner's lunge only your back knee is on the ground. Keep both hands on the ground inside your front leg. From this position, you're going to twist your upper back by raising your left arm up and over your head, keeping your right hand planted on the floor. Bring your left hand back to the floor, and repeat twice more on that side. Then step back to plank position, and repeat the movement three times on the right side. *This is the end of the flow sequence.*

REPEAT THIS WHOLE sequence up to three times until your body is warm and your joints feel juicy.

MENOPAUSE METABOLIC RESISTANCE (MMR) WORKOUTS

PHASE 1: MMR WORKOUTS 1, 2, AND 3

Phase 1 of the workouts is perfect for the ultimate beginner, restarter, or cardio queen looking to supplement her endurance training. You will stay with MMR Phase 1 for four to six weeks before moving on to Phase 2. All of the exercises are described in the Workout Exercise Library, beginning on page 191.

MMR 1

- Perform 8–10 reps (unless otherwise stated) of each exercise, moving in a circuit
- At the end of the circuit, rest for 1–2 minutes
- Do 2–4 rounds of each circuit

- Goblet Squat
- Pushup or Elevated Pushup
- Overhead Press
- Plank: no reps here, just hold for a minimum of 30 seconds
- Curtsy Lunge

MMR 2

- Perform 8–10 reps (unless otherwise stated) of each exercise, moving in a circuit
- At the end of the circuit, rest for 1–2 minutes
- Do 2–4 rounds of each circuit

- Romanian Deadlift
- Dead Bug: 5 slow reps on each side
- Floor Chest Press
- Reverse Lunge: do full reps on each leg
- Bent-Over Row

MMR 3

- Perform 8–10 reps (unless otherwise stated) of each exercise, moving in a circuit
- At the end of the circuit, rest for 1–2 minutes
- Do 2–4 rounds of each circuit

- Staggered Squat: do full reps on each leg
- Glute Bridge
- Bear Hover: hold for a minimum of 30 seconds
- Side Plank (regular or modified)
- Thruster

PHASE 2: MMR WORKOUTS 4, 5, AND 6

If you're feeling strong enough from Phase 1, then you're ready to kick it up a notch into Phase 2, where the exercises become progressively harder. Stay with Phase 2 for four to six weeks or until you feel strong enough to progress to Phase 3.

MMR 4

- Perform 8–12 reps (unless otherwise stated) of each exercise, moving in a circuit
- At the end of the circuit, rest for 1–2 minutes
- Do 3–5 rounds of each circuit

- Single-Leg Deadlift: do full reps on each leg
- Pushup or Elevated Pushup
- Thruster
- Jump Squat
- Bent-Over Row

MMR 5

- Perform 8–12 reps (unless otherwise stated) of each exercise, moving in a circuit
- At the end of the circuit, rest for 1–2 minutes
- Do 3–5 rounds of each circuit

- Goblet Squat
- Windmill: 5 reps on each side
- Clean: 15 reps
- Lateral Lunge: do full reps on each leg
- Renegade Row: do full reps on each side

MMR 6

- Perform 8–12 reps (unless otherwise stated) of each exercise, moving in a circuit
- At the end of the circuit, rest for 1–2 minutes
- Do 3–5 rounds of each circuit

- Single-Leg Glute Bridge: do full reps on each leg
- Bear Crawl: 45 seconds
- Curtsy Lunge: do full reps on each leg
- Up-Down plank: do full reps on each side
- Swing

PHASE 3: MMR WORKOUTS 7, 8, AND 9

By now you've been working out with me for over two months—go you! I know if you've followed Phase 1 and Phase 2 of the program, you will already be seeing significant gains in your strength. Phase 3 takes those strength gains and pushes your limits just a little bit more. Have fun with these workouts!

MMR 7

- Perform 8–12 reps (unless otherwise stated) of each exercise, moving in a circuit
- At the end of the circuit, rest for 1–2 minutes
- Do 3–5 rounds of each circuit

- Romanian Deadlift
- Floor Chest Press
- Side Plank: 45 to 60 seconds on each side
- Bent-Over Row
- Skater Jump: do full reps on each side

MMR 8

- Perform 8–12 reps (unless otherwise stated) of each exercise, moving in a circuit
- At the end of the circuit, rest for 1–2 minutes
- Do 3–5 rounds of each circuit

- Bulgarian Split Squat: do full reps on each leg
- Pushup
- Bear Crawl: 60 seconds
- Swing: 15 reps
- Windmill: 5 reps on each side

MMR 9

- Perform 8–12 reps (unless otherwise stated) of each exercise, moving in a circuit
- At the end of the circuit, rest for 1–2 minutes
- Do 3–5 rounds of each circuit

- Single-Leg Squat: do full reps on each leg
- Forearm Plank: 60 seconds
- Overhead Press
- Clean: 15 reps
- Jump Squat

WORKOUT EXERCISE LIBRARY

BEAR HOVER

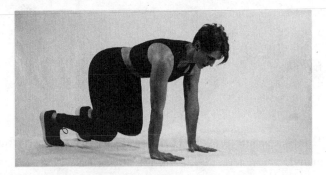

- This is essentially a plank but with your knees bent.

- Start on your hands and knees, engage your core, then let your knees float up from the floor around two inches.

- The aim is to maintain a normal spine, so don't let your butt poke up in the air. This will maintain a tight core.

- Push the floor away from you with both your toes and your hands.

- All of these cues will create a lot of tension in your body, so much so that you might be shaky after a few seconds. This is a good thing.

- Only hold the bear hover for as long as you can maintain both tension and great form, which won't be very long at first!

Pimp-It-Up Tip: Try a three-point bear hover. While keeping plenty of tension throughout the body, raise the right foot off the floor for a few seconds with control—keeping your foot flexed—then repeat on the left side.

BEAR CRAWL

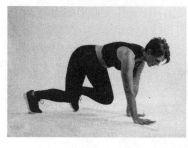 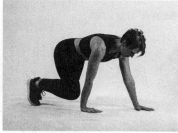

- The next logical step from the bear hover is the bear crawl.

- Start on your hands and knees, engage your core, and then let your knees float up from the floor around two inches.

- The aim is to maintain a normal spine, so don't let your butt poke up in the air. This will maintain a tight core.

- Lift your right hand and left foot simultaneously, and, with controlled movements, place them down a few inches in front. Then lift the left hand and right foot together. Start the crawl movement forward.

- Slow this exercise down; it will serve you better if you don't rush. You want to increase the *time under tension*, or the amount of time a muscle is under strain during a set.

Pimp-It-Up Tip: Change directions. Using the same deliberate control, move sideways, diagonally, and backward.

BENT-OVER ROW

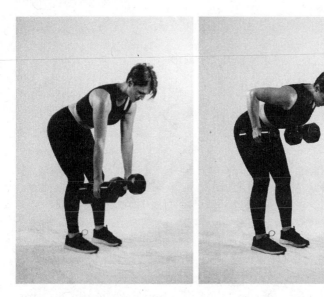

- Start in a hinged position (see Romanian Deadlift) with a set of dumbbells hanging down in front of your shins.

- Engage your core and keep your body still as you row the dumbbells up toward your rib cage, keeping your elbows relatively close to your body.

- Squeeze underneath your armpits to help engage your lats, keeping your shoulders away from your ears.

- Return to the starting position by lowering the dumbbells with control.

Pimp-It-Up Tip: You'll be surprised by how strong you are in this exercise, so don't be afraid to go heavy on the weights—your sexy back awaits you.

BULGARIAN SPLIT SQUAT

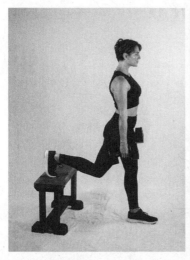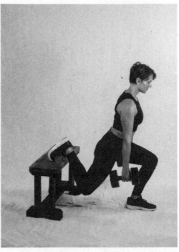

- Stand a few feet in front of a bench or chair, holding your dumbbells by your sides.

- Reach your right leg behind you and place it on the bench with your foot flat (upside down) or your toes curled under. My preference is to curl the toes under, but some people find that too unstable.

- Bend your left knee, taking your right knee toward the floor.

- In the lunge position your torso may lean slightly forward, but keep your chest lifted.

- Your front knee should be in line with your toes; make sure it doesn't fall inward.

- On an exhale push your left foot into the ground, using your foot to create stability, then push to standing.

- If your front heel lifts up, you need to move that foot forward slightly. Play around with the foot positions until this feels comfortable.

- Do all reps on one side before switching to the other.

Pimp-It-Up Tip: At the bottom of the movement you can increase the intensity of this exercise by adding a pulse. Straighten up your legs halfway, then dip back down again, before returning to starting position.

CLEAN

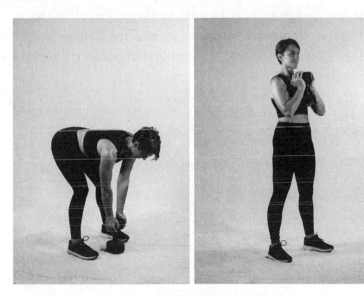

- Stand with feet slightly wider than your hips and one dumbbell standing upright on the floor between your legs. Your aim is to take the weight from the floor to your chest so that you end up holding the dumbbell in a "goblet" position. Don't spill your wine.

- Hinge at your hips (see Romanian Deadlift), bending the knees enough that you can grab the top of the dumbbell with both hands.

- Quickly drive your hips forward with power as you bring the dumbbell up the front of your body in a straight line and finally hold it in the goblet position.

- In the top position, tuck your elbows in slightly to support the dumbbell.

- Reverse the movement to lower the dumbbell.

Pimp-It-Up Tip: This can be a tricky exercise to get the hang of. Once you do, you'll want to go heavier. If more weight makes it hard to do with a dumbbell, consider trying this with a kettlebell.

CURTSY LUNGE

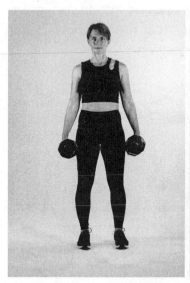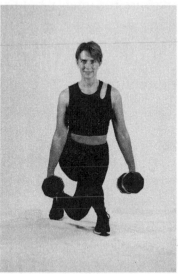

- Stand with feet slightly wider than your hips, holding both dumbbells by your sides.

- Take a deep breath in and engage your core, as you cross your left leg behind your right leg and bend both knees. Apparently this isn't how you would curtsy to the Queen of England, but imagine that's what you're doing!

- In the lunge position your torso should be straight and both hips aimed toward the front of the room; don't rotate your body.

- On an exhale, push your left foot into the ground, using your front foot to create stability, and return to standing.

- Do all reps on one side before switching to the other.

Pimp-It-Up Tip: At the bottom of the movement you can increase the intensity of this exercise by adding a pulse. Straighten up your legs halfway, then dip back down again, before returning to starting position.

DEAD BUG

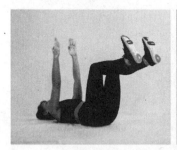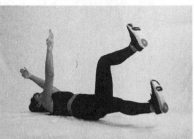

- Lie on the floor with your legs up, your knees bent at ninety degrees, and your arms raised straight above your chest. You want to keep your lower back in contact with the floor as much as possible. This should help you brace your core.

- While maintaining tension in your core, extend your left arm backward over your head while simultaneously extending your right leg straight out toward the floor, hovering about two inches from the ground. Make sure your foot remains flexed.

- If you are unable to lower your straight leg to the floor because you lack core strength or your lower back keeps lifting, then instead lower your heel and tap it on the floor with your knee bent.

- This is a super slow exercise, so you will perform fewer repetitions but with more time under tension, which refers to the time a muscle is under strain during a set. Done correctly, this should feel hard.

- Reverse the movement and switch to the other side, right arm overhead and left leg extended. Alternate sides.

Pimp-It-Up Tip: You can add intensity by holding a single dumbbell in both hands and taking that overhead as you extend each leg toward the floor.

ELEVATED PUSHUP

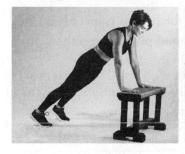 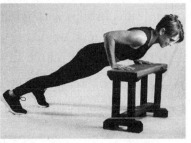

- Start in a straight-arm plank position with your hands on an elevated surface. This could be a kitchen counter-top, your workout bench, or a staircase. Play around until you find what works for you.

- Your hands should be positioned underneath your shoulders, and your body should be in a straight line from the top of your head to the heels of your feet. Lift your chin a little, so that you're looking slightly ahead of you rather than directly down at your hands.

- Take a deep breath in, engage your core, and actively engage your hands as if you're trying to pick up the surface.

- Maintaining tension throughout your body, lower yourself toward the elevated surface, maintaining the plank position at all times. In the bottom position your elbows should be pointing back at a forty-five-degree angle, not winging out to the sides.

- On an exhale drive your hands and toes actively into the ground and return to the plank position.

- If you cannot lower down toward the elevated surface, work on holding a straight-arm plank for at least forty-five seconds.

- Only do pushups with good form. If you can only do one good pushup, then do one good pushup and then work on holding your plank. Build up slowly.

Pimp-It-Up Tip: If you really find elevated pushups easy, then it's time to try full pushups. Good luck.

FLOOR CHEST PRESS

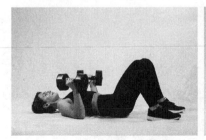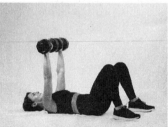

- Lie on your back with your knees bent and your feet flat on the floor. Hold a set of dumbbells at your chest with elbows bent, with your upper arms and elbows resting on the floor close to your body.

- Try to prevent your lower back from arching.

- Engage your core as you actively push into your heels and press the dumbbells straight up above your chest, finding a hand position that works best for you.

- Keep your elbows in close, so that the weight doesn't stray away from the body.

- Return the dumbbells to start position.

Pimp-It-Up Tip: This is a lot harder than it looks, as you have no momentum to help you lift the weight. To make this even harder, do the exercise with one arm at a time, which requires you to use more core to control the movement.

FOREARM PLANK

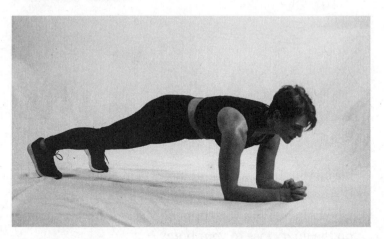

- Lie on your front. Place your forearms on the floor at right angles to your shoulders. Interlace your fingers in front of you.

- Lift yourself up off the floor, balanced on your forearms and your toes. Your body should make a straight line from the top of your head to your heels. Lift your chin a little so that you're looking slightly ahead rather than directly down at the floor.

- Squeeze your bum cheeks, as if I'm trying to pull a $100 bill from the crack. Engage your core hard, like you're bracing for a punch. (I know these cues are crazy, but they work!)

- Push the floor away from you with both your toes and your forearms, and squeeze your hands together.

- All of these cues will create a lot of tension in your body, so much so that you might be shaky after a few seconds. This is a good thing.

- Only hold the plank for as long as you can maintain both tension and great form, which won't be very long!

Pimp-It-Up Tip: Try three-point forearm planks. While keeping plenty of tension throughout your body, lift your right foot off the floor for a few seconds, with control, keeping your foot flexed. Then repeat on the left side.

GLUTE BRIDGE

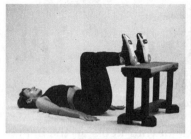 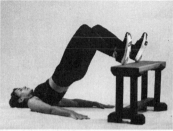

- You'll need a chair or bench for this exercise.

- Lie on your back, and place your heels up on the bench with knees bent. Keep your arms on the ground with palms pushing into the floor.

- Engage your core as you actively push into your heel and lift your butt up off the ground.

- At the top of the movement, you should be resting on the tops of your shoulders, and there should be a straight line from the tops of your knees to the tips of your shoulders.

- Reverse the movement by lowering your hips.

Pimp-It-Up Tip: At the top of the movement, focus on a tight squeeze of your butt. You can increase the intensity of this exercise by adding a pulse. At the top of the exercise lower your hips slightly, then lift again before returning to starting position.

SINGLE-LEG GLUTE BRIDGE

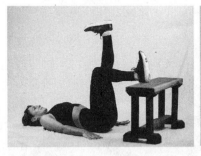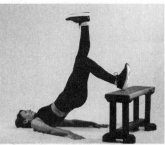

- You'll need a chair or bench for this exercise.

- Lie on your back. Place one of your heels on the bench with your knee bent, point the other leg up into the air, and keep your arms on the ground with palms pushing into the floor. Your extended leg can be slightly bent.

- Engage your core as you actively push into the heel on the bench and lift up your butt, squeezing it tightly.

- At the top of the movement, you should be resting on the tops of your shoulders and there should be a straight line from your knees to your shoulders.

- This exercise makes you feel very unstable, so take your time and use your core strength to control the movement.

- Reverse the movement by lowering your hips.

- Do all reps on one side before switching to the other.

Pimp-It-Up Tip: This is a challenging exercise, but if you want to make it even more challenging try straightening your extended leg. This increases the length of the lever and makes it harder to keep your balance, which in turn means you have to engage both your core and butt even more.

GOBLET SQUAT

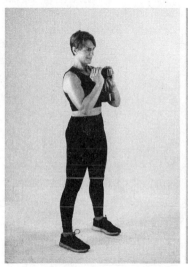 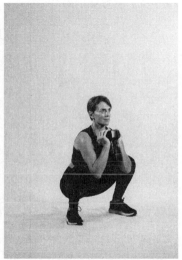

- Stand with your feet slightly wider than your hips, holding one dumbbell in front of your chest like a goblet of wine.

- Take a deep breath in and engage your core, then bend your knees as if you're sitting down, taking your bum toward the floor.

- You may need to adjust your feet wider or narrower to feel comfortable in this position. Turning your toes outward can be helpful.

- On an exhale push your feet into the ground and your knees out slightly as you return to standing.

Pimp-It-Up Tip: You can increase the intensity of this exercise by pausing at the bottom of the exercise for three seconds.

JUMP SQUAT

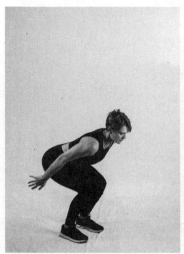 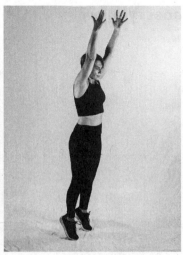

- Stand with your feet slightly wider than your hips, with your arms by your sides. Bend your knees to a low squat position.

- Using your arms to drive the movement upward, push away from the floor as you jump up as high as you can.

- Land like a cat, as quietly as possible, back into a low squat and repeat the movement.

- Make sure your knees stay in alignment with your toes and don't fall inward on this exercise.

- You may need to adjust your feet wider or narrower to feel comfortable in this position.

Pimp-It-Up Tip: You can increase the intensity of this exercise by holding a set of dumbbells. Rather than use your arms to propel the movement, you are adding a resisting force by keeping the dumbbells at your side.

LATERAL LUNGE

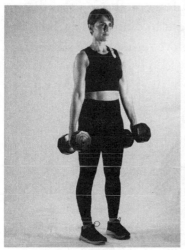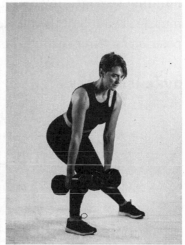

- Stand with your feet slightly wider than your hips, holding both dumbbells by your sides.

- Take a deep breath in and engage your core as you take a big step out to the side with your right leg. As you place your foot down, actively plant your right toes into the floor. Your dumbbells will hang directly on either side of your right knee.

- In the lunge position your right leg should be at a right angle, with your knee in line with your toes. Drive your butt back, like you're about to sit down on the loo. Your leg left can be straight or have a slight bend in the knee. Take your time to get the position right.

- On an exhale, drive your right foot into the ground as you push to standing.

- Do all reps on one side before switching to the other.

Pimp-It-Up Tip: This is all about working on balance and building strength in the gluteus medius, a stabilizing muscle in your butt. If you want to pimp this up, hold the position for three seconds before returning to standing.

OVERHEAD PRESS

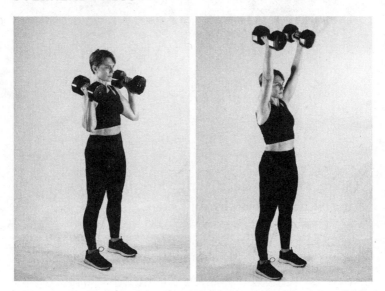

- Stand with your feet slightly wider than your hips, holding your dumbbells up at your shoulders.

- Take a deep breath in and engage your core, then as you breathe out, push your feet dynamically into the floor and raise the dumbbells overhead.

- Keep your body straight and don't push through your knees.

- You want this to be a strict press, which means that you push the weight straight from your shoulders and don't add any pre-movement momentum. You will find that engaging your core helps create strength through the movement.

- Lower the dumbbells back to shoulder height with control, and repeat.

Pimp-It-Up Tip: If you want a more dynamic move and the ability to lift a heavier weight, you can add a small push-press. Do this by slightly bending your knees and then pushing them straight, using the power of your legs to help drive the weight overhead.

PUSHUP

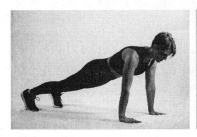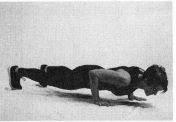

- Start in a straight-arm plank position, your hands positioned underneath your shoulders. Your body should be in a straight line from the top of your head to the heels of your feet. Lift your chin a little, so that you're looking slightly ahead of you rather than directly down at the floor.

- Take a deep breath in, engage your core, and actively engage your hands as if you're trying to pick up your mat.

- Maintaining tension throughout your body, lower yourself toward the floor, maintaining the plank position at all times. In the bottom position your elbows should be pointing back at a forty-five-degree angle, not winging out to the sides.

- On an exhale drive your hands and toes actively into the ground and return to the plank position.

- If you cannot lower down toward the floor, go back to the elevated pushup or work on holding a straight-arm plank for at least forty-five seconds.

- Only do pushups with good form. If you can only do one good pushup, then do one good pushup and then take it back down to either an elevated pushup or a plank exercise. Build up slowly.

Pimp-It-Up Tip: If you really find pushups easy, then *wow!* Good for you. Consider elevating your feet onto a bench for added resistance.

RENEGADE ROW

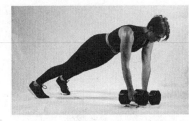 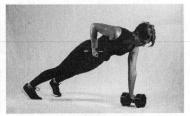

- Start in a straight-arm plank position, with your hands positioned underneath your shoulders holding onto a set of dumbbells.

- Your body should be in a straight line from the top of your head to your heels. Lift your chin a little, so that you're looking slightly ahead of you rather than directly down at the floor.

- Take a deep breath in and engage your core, as you row the dumbbell on your right toward your rib cage, keeping your elbow relatively close to your body.

- Keep your hips facing toward the floor; you are actively trying to resist any rotation of the body.

- On an exhale lower the weight toward the floor and return to the plank position.

- Only do renegade rows with good form. If you need to, try this exercise without a weight or stick with the plank exercise until you build up strength. Be patient.

- Alternate sides.

Pimp-It-Up Tip: This is a hard exercise at the best of times, but if you want to increase the intensity, simply add five more reps on each side.

REVERSE LUNGE

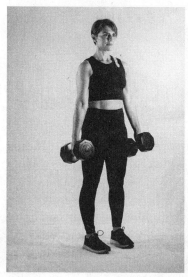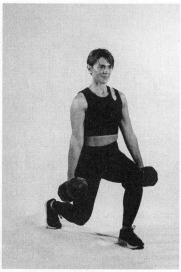

- Stand with your feet slightly wider than your hips, holding both dumbbells by your sides.

- Take a deep breath in and engage your core. Take your right leg and step it behind you, actively planting your right toes into the floor. Bend your legs, aiming your back knee toward the floor.

- In the lunge position, both your back leg and your front leg should be bent at a ninety-degree angle. This matters, so take your time to get the position right.

- On an exhale, push your back foot into the ground, using your front foot to create stability; then push to standing.

- Do all reps on one side before switching to the other.

Pimp-It-Up Tip: I always start people working with the reverse lunge, as it helps in understanding balance and control. If you feel good doing the reverse lunge, then pimp it up by trying the forward lunge. But remember: form matters.

ROMANIAN DEADLIFT

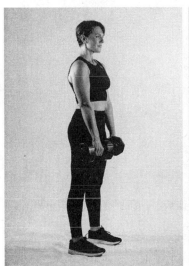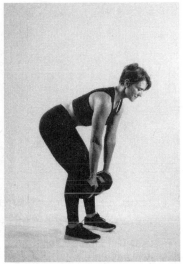

- Start in a tall standing position with the dumbbells resting on the tops of your thighs.

- Keep your head and chest lifted as you hinge your hips back, keeping a slight bend in your knees. Keep the dumbbells really close to your body, almost as if they are drawing a line down your leg.

- Hinge to your full range of motion, ideally reaching the dumbbells to the level of your shins. At this stage you should feel your hamstrings scream out for mercy.

- Return to starting position by pushing your feet into the ground and driving your hips forward—give a good old thrust!

Pimp-It-Up Tip: You'll be surprised by how strong you are in this exercise, so don't be afraid to go heavy on the weights—your butt will thank you.

SIDE PLANK

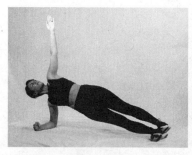 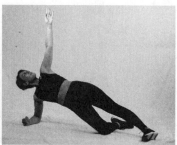

- Lie on your right side with your feet stacked on top of each other and your elbow lined up underneath your shoulder.

- Make a fist with your right hand, which will create tension and support the right shoulder joint.

- Push up from the floor so that you're supporting your body weight on your forearm and feet.

- Keep your body in a straight line from your head to your feet; resist the urge to lean forward or back in this exercise.

- To modify this exercise, it's perfectly acceptable to put your right knee on the floor until you build up enough strength to extend both legs.

- Your left hand can rest on your hip or you can point it upward, which will add to the challenge of maintaining your balance.

- Complete on one side before switching to the other.

Pimp-It-Up Tip: If you can successfully hold a side plank for forty-five seconds, then work toward a leg lift, holding the top leg away from the bottom leg for as long as you can stand it.

SINGLE-LEG DEADLIFT

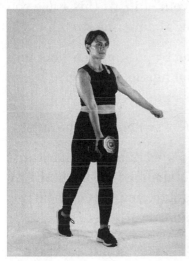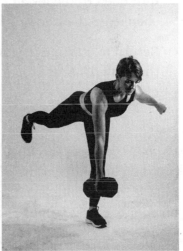

- There are so many variations of this exercise that you need to find the level that suits you best.

  › Beginners: take one leg backward like a kick-stand, but don't take it off the floor.

  › Intermediate: do this using your body weight only.

> › Advanced: use a dumbbell in the opposite hand from your working leg.

- Start in a tall standing position. Put 80 percent of your weight on your front foot and actively ground that foot into the floor.

- With a slight bend in your standing knee, keep your head and chest lifted, then hinge your hips back, lifting your back leg off the floor. Keep your hips facing the floor; don't open them up to the sky.

- Hinge to your full range of motion, ideally reaching the dumbbell to the level of your shin. At this stage you should feel the standing leg's hamstring stretch.

- Return to starting position by pushing your foot into the ground and driving your hips forward—give a good old thrust!

- Do all reps on one side before switching to the other.

Pimp-It-Up Tip: This is all about working on balance and building strength in the gluteus medius, a stabilizing muscle in your butt. If you want to pimp this up, hold this position for three seconds before returning to standing.

SINGLE-LEG SQUAT

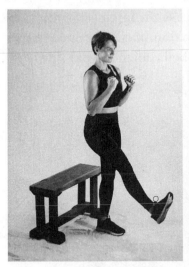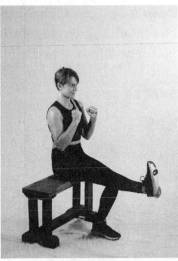

- You'll need a chair or bench for this exercise. Position yourself so that you can sit back safely onto it.

- This is more achievable if your feet are close together. Lift one leg and extend it in front of you, either elevated off the ground or with the heel touching the floor.

- Bend your standing leg, and sit back toward the bench behind you. All the time engage your core and think about squeezing your inner thighs together. Sit right down on the bench.

- Don't worry if you find it hard to get up; it is! (And you're not allowed to use your hands.) On an exhale, engage your core and plant that standing foot hard into the ground. Squeeze your inner thighs tightly together as you push yourself back to starting position.

- Do all reps on one side before switching to the other.

Pimp-It-Up Tip: You can increase the intensity of this exercise by adding weight. Hold a dumbbell at your chest in a goblet position or two dumbbells down by your sides.

SKATER JUMP

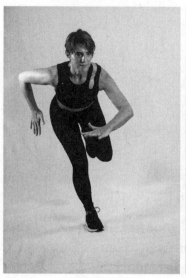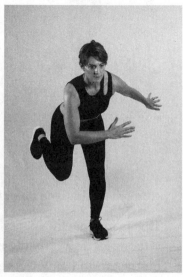

- From standing, shift your weight onto your right leg. Position your left leg behind the right, with the foot on the floor or raised in the air.

- Jump to the left, landing on your left foot only. Cross your right foot behind the left knee, either touching it lightly on the floor or balancing it in the air.

- Repeat the movement to the right side.

- Use your arms for propulsion to drive the movement from side to side.

- To modify this exercise, you can step from side to side rather than jump. As you get stronger, add the dynamic jump and increase the speed.

Pimp-It-Up Tip: You can increase the intensity of this exercise by holding a set of dumbbells by your sides.

STAGGERED SQUAT

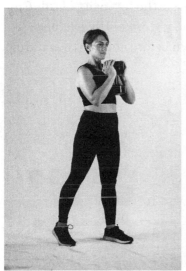
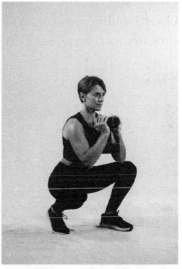

- Stagger your stance so that your left foot is forward and your right foot is back, holding a dumbbell in front of your chest like a goblet of wine.

- Take a deep breath in and engage your core, then bend your knees like you're sitting down, taking your bum toward the floor.

- Keep your front foot flat on the floor, and come onto the toes of your rear foot. Approximately 80 percent of your weight will be on your front leg.

- You may need to adjust your feet wider or narrower to feel comfortable in this position. Turning your toes outward can be helpful.

- On an exhale, push your feet into the ground and your knees out slightly as you return to standing.

- Do all reps on one side before switching to the other.

Pimp-It-Up Tip: You can increase the intensity of this exercise by adding a pulse. At the bottom of the exercise, rise up halfway, then go back down before coming to standing.

SWING

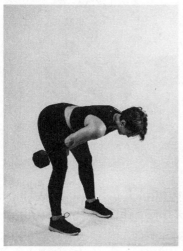 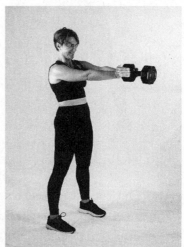

- Stand with your feet slightly wider than your hips. Place a single dumbbell upright on the floor, slightly in front of you.

- Pick up the dumbbell with two hands. Holding it securely, swing it back between your legs, pushing your bum back in a hinge position (see the Romanian Dead-lift); your forearms should hit the inside of your legs.

- Now comes the tricky part, so pay attention! When the dumbbell reaches its farthest point behind you, stand up as quickly as you can by thrusting your hips forward and keeping your arms straight.

- The dumbbell should shoot up with the momentum of this movement until it reaches shoulder height.

- As the dumbbell starts to fall back down, let it swing back between your legs with control.

- This is a very dynamic movement. You are not lifting the dumbbell; rather it is being thrust up by the power of your hip hinge.

- At the top of the movement, your body should resemble a standing plank. That is, you should be in a straight line from head to feet, with your butt clenched and your core engaged.

Pimp-It-Up Tip: This exercise is best performed with a kettlebell, so if you have access to one, then you can go heavier.

THRUSTER

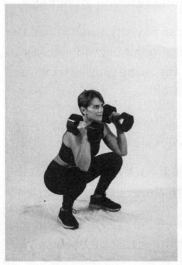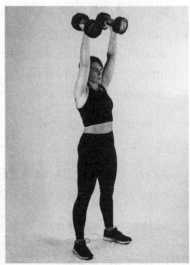

- Stand with feet slightly wider than your hips, holding your dumbbells at your shoulders.

- Take a deep breath in, engage your core, and bend your knees to a low squat.

- You may need to adjust your feet wider or narrower to feel comfortable in this position. Turning your toes outward can be helpful.

- As you breathe out, push your feet dynamically into the floor and power the dumbbells overhead.

- The momentum of the thrust up from the squat should push the weights up easily.

- Lower the dumbbells back to shoulder height, with control, and repeat.

Pimp-It-Up Tip: Add challenge to the exercise by staggering your feet (see Staggered Squat) to create some instability, making you work a little harder to perform the exercise.

UP-DOWN PLANK

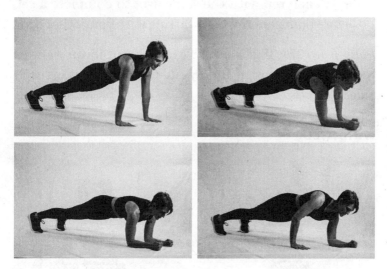

- Start in a straight-arm plank position, your hands positioned underneath your shoulders, with hands and feet actively pushing into the ground.

- Lower your right elbow to the mat and then your left, coming into a forearm plank. Take this moment to recheck your form.

- Put your right hand on the mat and straighten your right elbow. Do the same on the left to return to a full plank.

- Don't rock! Keep your hips facing toward the floor; you are actively trying to resist any rotation of the body.

- Only do up-down planks with good form. If this is too hard for you, decrease the number of reps on each side or stick with the plank exercise until you build up strength. Be patient.

- Start each rep with the same arm to complete a set, before doing another set starting with your other arm.

Pimp-It-Up Tip: This is a hard exercise, but if you want to increase the intensity, simply add five more reps on each side.

WINDMILL

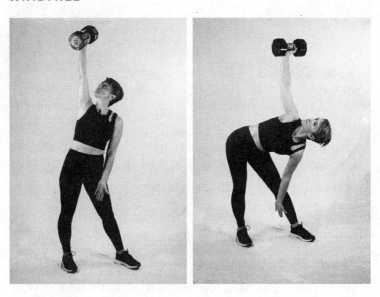

- With feet slightly wider than your hips, point both feet to the left. With a dumbbell in your right hand, raise your arm overhead. Place your left hand on the inside of your left thigh and look up at the dumbbell.

- Take your time with the setup and play around with the foot position until you feel comfortable.

- Keeping most of your weight on your right leg, push your hips out to the right side and keep the weight overhead pointing toward the ceiling. Your right leg and your right arm stay straight.

- Bend down to the left. Use your left hand to track along the inside of your left leg until you can feel a good stretch in your hamstrings.

- Push both feet into the floor and drive the dumbbell up toward the ceiling as you return to standing.

- Do all reps on one side before switching to the other.

- Start with a lighter weight until you get the form nailed down, then move up to a more challenging weight.

Pimp-It-Up Tip: Take a small child and raise it over your head, following all cues for the windmill exercise. Okay, okay, just kidding. The best way to make this exercise harder is to slow down the movement and/or add more weight.

A SAMPLE WEEKLY SCHEDULE

Here's an example of how you might schedule your workouts over a two-week period:

- Move through your three workouts over the week: MMR 1, MMR 2, then MMR 3. Do the workouts in this order even if you miss a workout session (for example, if you miss MMR 2 on Wednesday, don't just skip to MMR 3;

instead, do MMR 2 on your next scheduled day, and shift all workouts accordingly).

- Aim for two to four MMR workouts a week—three is ideal.

- You need at least three NEAT sessions a week. Prioritize your active recovery. Walking is clearly the easiest way to make this happen; aiming for 6,000 to 8,000 steps is a good goal. Other ideas include yoga, swimming, cycling, mowing the lawn, and shoveling snow (thankfully I don't need to do that here in Texas).

- Continue rotating through the three workouts of the phase you're in for about four to six weeks. Move on to the next phase when you feel ready.

	MON	TUE	WED	THU	FRI	SAT	SUN
WEEK 1	MMR 1	NEAT	MMR 2	NEAT	MMR 3	OFF	NEAT
WEEK 2	MMR 1	NEAT	NEAT	MMR 2	OFF	MMR 3	NEAT

Note: I used to get frustrated if I lost three days of my workout plan to utter fatigue or migraines. Now I just accept that these changes are going to happen, and I alter my workout to suit my needs. You can do this by replacing an MMR session with NEAT, by doing the dynamic warm-up sequence, or by reducing the weights in your MMR workout, focusing on form instead of pushing to your usual level of fatigue. Being adaptable is paramount! The important thing about working out during menopause is to accept how your body feels. You're going to have really shitty days, but they won't last forever. Just jump back in as soon as you feel capable, without any judgment.

I HOPE THAT after reading this chapter you're as excited about strength training as I am. I know one of the major stumbling blocks for women is getting started. It can feel intimidating and confusing (once I was followed around the gym by a newbie who copied every exercise I did—in the end I wrote her out a program of her own). I get it. We're all beginners at some stage. These workouts have been developed to help introduce you to the world of weights and to help seasoned professionals get some structure back into their schedule. This is meant to be fun, ladies, not a pain in the arse. Set yourself up for success by adopting these strategic hacks.

MMR

- Aim for three MMR workouts a week.

- Keep the workouts short and intense.

- Only work out when you feel that your energy levels are right.

- If you're too fatigued to work out, wait until the next day.

NEAT

- Go for a relaxing walk, especially outside in nature.

- Do some housework. You'll be surprised how many calories that burns.

- Get off the bus or train a stop earlier and walk the remainder of your journey.

- Swim, go for a bike ride, do yoga or Zumba, wiggle your hips and get juicy with joy, or run around with your dog or your kids.

HOW TO DE-STRESS (CALM THE EFF DOWN!) AND GET SOME SLEEP

B OY, HAVE MY eyes been opened to stress during the menopocalypse. I have always been a bit fiery, never afraid to speak my mind and stand up for myself in an argument, but I also haven't actively sought out conflict. During my menopause journey, however, shit got crazy! There was a stage where I just wanted to argue with anybody and everybody, even my own reflection. I am all about keeping it real with my family—they see the full spectrum of everything I'm experiencing. But there were times, especially in perimenopause, where the stress got hold of me in a way that I just couldn't control.

One day, I was in the kitchen with the kids when my older son said something that pushed my buttons as only a teenager can. I turned around and screamed in his face like a wild banshee. I was out of control: I said horrible things that I didn't mean, I scared him, and I was utterly ashamed of myself. I could feel my heart pumping and my temperature rising.

Although the incident was short-lived, and my son seemed to recover quite quickly, I didn't. I couldn't let go of the shame of treating him so badly. And the burden of feeling this heavy stress in my body was exhausting me. I was in a terrible cycle of being fiery toward my family and then depressed by my actions, on repeat.

That incident was another one of those light-bulb moments where I realized I had to do something. I couldn't carry on feeling that way and expecting my family to keep understanding and being tolerant.

Stress shows itself in a multitude of ways that are not always apparent. We often say that we feel stressed, or that something was stressful, but do you truly understand what it means when your body is stressed, especially through menopause?

WHAT IS STRESS?

Simply stated, stress is the body's way of responding to a demand or a threat. It is the body's automatic reaction to those events to protect you, which means that cortisol isn't always the bad guy.

Our bodies are actually built to handle some stress: I'm guessing you're familiar with the phrase "fight or flight or freeze" (AKA the stress response). This is the physiological process that kicks in if you're feeling threatened, whether the impending threat is physical, mental, or emotional. This automatic response includes feeling alert, responsive, and focused, which can be lifesaving in some threatening situations. It can also help you rise to a challenge by improving your concentration and boosting your courage in a challenging moment, which is also a great tie-in to the previous chapter, on strength training—the two go hand-in-hand. Being moved beyond our comfort zone at times—through a stressful situation or through challenging exercise—helps us grow and appreciate our own resilience. We are tough! We've all been through challenges, but we survived and are stronger.

Now here's the kicker: your body doesn't distinguish between these two scenarios. It doesn't matter to your body if the response is to something real or perceived; it's just designed to respond rapidly. The hormonal response is going to be the same if the threat is real (you're about to be eaten by a lion) or perceived (somebody disagrees with your viewpoint; this might feel like a real threat but that's just how you perceive it. We've all been in social media battles that dent our ego. But they're not threats to our lives). We get stressed when there's a disconnect between the situation and the resources (energy) available to handle it. If we don't handle stress appropriately, our brains and bodies get taxed to the point where mental health and physical problems can arise, such as depression, anxiety, and heart disease.

· Your adrenal glands are responsible for producing cortisol, which is known as the stress hormone. During menopause, we experience higher levels of cortisol in our system as a result of fluctuations in our other hormones—surprise, surprise. Progesterone, if you remember from Chapter 1, has a calming effect on the body, But as our progesterone levels start to decline, we have less of a buffer against cortisol and therefore are less able to tolerate stress than we were pre-menopause. I find this a little reassuring: at least there's a reason for the erratic mood swings, and eventually the hormone levels will calm down, as will we.

There is *good* stress. Excitement over an upcoming event, exhilaration after a good workout, or the thrill of accepting a new challenge—these are all good feelings. They all might feel a little scary or new, but that doesn't last long, or it's intermittent, and afterward you feel great. It's a bit like riding a rollercoaster. We've all had those feelings of excitement mixed with dread at the thought of what is coming, but afterward we feel invigorated. It's the type of stress that we want to experience in our lives.

During menopause women often report losing that good-stress feeling, and at the same time feeling more of the bad stress, which is the kind that stays around longer and is harder to recover from. Our fluctuating sex hormones make it harder for us to cope with everyday stress, so during menopause we have to actively look at ways to help manage it.

I recently went boogie boarding in Los Angeles with some friends. Before I got in the water I felt a little apprehension (a little bit of that good stress), but I still went ahead and tried it. The water was choppy and thrilling. I fell in, I laughed, I swallowed too much water, and afterward I felt on top of the world. It was so much fun. It's really important for us to find those moments in life that make us truly thrive.

Good and bad stress both have a profound effect on your body. Good stress is short-term, helps to keep us alert, serves as a positive influence, and motivates us to give our all. When you have a deadline at work, for example, good stress can temporarily help boost your brain power and put you in a heightened state of awareness. This type of situation, whether at work, in sports, or during the creative process, can help you be accountable for your actions and motivate you to be a better person. With the right amount of *good stress*, you can really thrive.

In contrast, living with *bad stress* can be detrimental to your health. High levels of cortisol can affect your quality of sleep and increase body fat. Chronic, long-term stress can lead to serious health issues such as heart disease, depression, and anxiety, which can be extremely difficult to recover from. That's why menopausal women need to actively seek out relaxation, through activities like meditation, walking, yoga, or mindfulness. These kinds of activities help to kick-start the parasympathetic nervous system, which counteracts the "fight or flight or freeze" response and is involved in recuperation, digestion, and recovery. You have to find time during menopause to reduce the stress burden on your body, because it simply won't happen on its own.

Here's an easy way to identify the difference between good stress and bad stress:

- Good stress is short-lived and infrequent.

- Bad stress is chronic and hinders your everyday life.

Other independent risk factors for stress during menopause include poor sleep due to fluctuating hormones (yes, poor sleep causes stress and stress causes poor sleep!), negative life events, lack of employment, change in family dynamics, and the natural aging process, which can certainly contribute to higher levels of stress and even depression. It's all connected. It's important to recognize the deep biochemical changes associated with such events and the impact they have on your body.

SYMPTOMS OF STRESS

Do you recognize any of the symptoms listed below? I certainly do, and the ironic thing is that most of the symptoms of stress are identical to the symptoms of menopause. Stress is a big part of menopause, and menopausal symptoms feel much worse when you are stressed out to the hilt.

- Insomnia

- Low energy, even if you're getting adequate sleep

- Frequent colds

- Cravings for unhealthful foods

- Digestion problems like bloating

- Weight gain, especially around the middle

- Low libido

- More aches and pains

- Low mood, irritability

- Anxiety and depression

MENOPAUSE AND STRESS

Menopause puts us in a bewildering and upsetting new environment. You have a new body to deal with. You have all the changes of middle age, from becoming an empty nester to being part of the squeeze generation to juggling your career and planning your future. These changes all cause emotional, physical, and mental stress, which leaves its effects on your body. If you don't take the time to manage these stresses, the resulting high levels of cortisol can affect your blood-sugar levels and cause a craving for carbs, which you most likely don't need and which then are deposited as fat.

As I have mentioned, your body doesn't perceive the difference between real and imaginary threats. If you're being chased by a saber-toothed tiger down the streets of L.A., your body will respond by going into survival mode because it really wants you to live. Fight-or-flight mode will kick in and your body will make glucose (via carbs) available for fuel so that you can either run away quickly or fight that fierce pussycat with all your might.

In real life there may be no saber-toothed tiger to run away from, but your body will still produce that fuel for you to use. Short-term stress will use the fuel efficiently; for example, when you have a deadline at the office it will help you bust through the paperwork and feel a sense of achievement. This type of everyday stress is normal, and the body can cope with it. Unfortunately, longer-term stresses like the loss of a loved one, depression, PTSD, being a long-term caregiver, or even an unhealthy lifestyle will constantly activate the body's stress-response system. This can put you in danger of becoming insulin-resistant, because you now have too much blood sugar in your system, making you more likely to store belly fat. (For a reminder of how this works, see the insulin and cortisol connection in Chapter 5.)

NUTRITION AND STRESS

This is why in addition to managing your stress levels in menopause, you must focus on nutrition. To ensure that you don't create spikes in your blood sugar, you must eat nutritious meals. Higher levels of blood sugar lead to increased fatigue, mood swings, and lapses in concentration, adding more stress to your body. When your body is stressed, you want to eat highly processed foods with extra fats and added sugars, but if you can focus on consuming protein and healthy fats to keep you satiated, and complex carbs to keep your blood-sugar levels stable, you will give your body a chance to calm the fook down.

This is also a reason I am not a fan of intermittent fasting and other fad diets for women during menopause. Extreme dieting and fasting can put your body under stress, and although at another time of life your body may have responded favorably to the diet, during menopause it's just not going to work. Fad diets that eliminate food groups prevent your body from getting all the nutrients it needs to function properly and manage stress.

I tried intermittent fasting in perimenopause and had disastrous results. I was constantly hungry, putting my body under more stress; I started putting weight on my tummy, as my body perceived a need to conserve fat; and I generally did not have any energy. Eating breakfast allowed me to feel satiated, fueled for my workouts, and less stressed. There are some women in my online community who have done well on intermittent fasting, but again this is a case of one size doesn't fit all. If you like eating breakfast, there's no reason to stop. If you don't get hungry until lunchtime, however, then intermittent fasting may work for you without being too stressful.

EXERCISE AND STRESS

More than ever it's going to be apparent to you that you need to schedule days to rest. Exercise can be a savior during menopause, but it can also become too much of a good thing. That's why my exercise program includes recovery days, which allow your body to recover from the demands of your workout days and can make a difference to your overall wellness.

Let's review. During menopause, hormonal changes put the body under much more stress than usual. From the harsh symptoms to the inability to cope emotionally, along with all the other midlife stresses we're already faced with, we sometimes feel like our body is betraying us. When we add additional stresses in the form of exercise, we have to allow our body to recover and regain its equilibrium.

We have become an all-or-nothing society. We have almost shamed ourselves into thinking that rest is wrong, that slowing down is bad. Well, it's not. Being intuitive and learning to understand the needs of your body will help you gain more strength and resilience. When you exercise, your body becomes stressed and releases cortisol, but you now know that too much cortisol is not a good thing. So how are you supposed to know how much stress your body can handle?

Every time you work out, you are creating micro-tears in your muscle fibers, which are necessary for your muscles to grow. Without damage (a stimulus), there can be no response from the body. Your body expects this and, in fact, craves this adaptation, and you can aid the process with rest and good nutrition to fuel the recovery. It's very difficult to create this type of stimulus with long, steady cardio or bodyweight exercises like calisthenics and yoga, which is why it's so important to have a strength-based program in your arsenal. Doing a strength-based workout three times a week is what we are aiming for, and you must balance that with adequate rest and recovery days.

A 2012 study by the Technical University of Dresden, Germany, showed that longer endurance sessions deplete your energy stores and release more cortisol, whereas short, more intense strength workouts, like the MMRs in this book, cause less of an increase in cortisol production, providing that you rest between exercises.

Strength training will make your body more efficient at managing glucose and reduce your stress. Your lower stress levels will in turn help keep your cortisol levels in check so that you won't have terrible spikes in your blood sugar and then that rotten crashing fatigue that follows it. Combining this with active rest days actually allows you to become kick-ass strong and resilient in menopause. In Chapter 8, I gave you a schedule for your workouts that specifically asks you to do active rest days. These can be fun and interesting and they are not optional.

MINDFULNESS AND BREATHING

It wasn't until an endocrinologist named Hans Selye identified biological stress in the late 1950s that people started delving deeper and doing research into stress. Obviously biological stress has always been around, but Selye's discovery has probably helped millions of people to cope with stress every day. Thank you, Hans!

Unless you're taking HT, there's very little you can do to control your sex hormones, so estrogen and progesterone are going to keep spiking and falling for a number of years no matter what you do. What you can control is your cortisol, and this hormone can be directly affected by the things you do. Making choices that help reduce your cortisol should be your priority.

Let's start with mindfulness. In the past when I heard that term, I envisaged some hippie-type sage chanting "ohm" in some ridiculous yoga position, but this is an outdated view. Mindfulness is simply the ability to be fully present, aware of where you are and what you are doing and not reacting to or being overwhelmed by what's going on around you.

How often can you say that you are being truly mindful? We often get so distracted or overwhelmed by what's going on around us and the thoughts in our own minds that we truly can't just be in the present moment. Mindfulness practice can look different to everybody. For some people it is a prescribed meditation while sitting, walking, or lying down, but for others it can just mean being aware of and controlling their experiences and emotions.

I require stillness. I'm a very active person who rarely sits, but I have often found myself needing to just stop and take stock. This never happened before I started perimenopause; I never felt the need. Now every day I take my cup of morning coffee outside (living in Texas, I enjoy permanent good weather!), and sit quietly for five minutes. I don't focus on anything, I don't think about anything, I simply take in nature and relax. If thoughts come into my head, I acknowledge them but don't let them stay. This simple step has helped keep me sane, but it did take me some time to feel comfortable doing it. It didn't come easily to me, but I knew it was worth the perseverance.

It is well documented that conscious breathing helps alleviate stress by reducing anxiety and pressing a big reset button on your mind. As we discussed in Chapter 4, your diaphragm is your breathing muscle, located just under your ribcage. I often see people breathing directly into their chest area and taking short stressful breaths— there's nothing relaxing about that at all. When you breathe with your diaphragm, you breathe deeply enough to push your ribcage out sideways and fill your belly with air. If you are feeling overwhelmed, angry, or anxious, try the box-breathing technique described in Chapter 4. It feels fantastic, I promise you, and it keeps your pelvic floor in check too!

My son has had success with cognitive behavioral therapy (CBT) techniques, and a large component of that practice is integrating his breathing technique into stressful situations. Rather than react to the stress, he stops and focuses on taking deep breaths, eliciting a calming response in his nervous system. It's a very useful technique to have in your toolbox.

Some other things you might want to try to reduce stress are: meditating, reading, talking to a friend, listening to music, drinking tea, taking a nap (if your schedule allows—and yeah, I could sometimes nap twice a day), exercising, going for a walk, or even just taking the time to reframe the situation. If you're worried about something specific, think about the possible positive outcomes of the situation or how you might approach it from a different viewpoint. I encourage you to spend as much energy as you can on the things that help you decompress so that you can put things into perspective.

THE IMPORTANCE OF SLEEP

Has your sleep been affected by menopause? Sleep quality in general starts to deteriorate with age. With the added complexity of menopause, more than 50 percent of women peri- to postmenopause report difficulties with sleeping. Disruptions from hot flashes, night sweats, apnea, insomnia, anxiety, and stress are all reasons that sleep may be disturbed. In some circumstances, medical intervention may be necessary, which could take the form of hormone therapy or prescription medication.

We also know that good-quality sleep is an integral part of fat loss—studies have linked fat gain with too little sleep (as well as with too much sleep!), because lack of sleep can trigger food cravings. Experts have determined that the minimum number of hours of sleep adults need for optimum weight loss and overall health is around seven hours each night.

MENOPAUSE AND INSOMNIA

It seems generally that postmenopausal women are the unhappiest about their sleep quality. The National Sleep Foundation reports that 61 percent of postmenopausal women suffer from insomnia. Progesterone and estrogen play a role in this, as both are conducive to sleep. Progesterone is known for its sedative effects and ability to reduce anxiety, and estrogen plays a number of roles, including regulating the number of times we wake up during the night, the amount of dream sleep (REM) we experience, and how long it takes us to fall asleep. When those hormones start to dwindle, we start experiencing major sleep disturbances.

You aren't wasting time during sleep. The body uses your sleeping hours to repair and rejuvenate, so it's crucial to your overall health. Chronically low sleep increases your likelihood of chronic illness, elevates your sympathetic nervous system response, decreases growth hormone (GH) and thyroid stimulating hormone (TSH), and increases cortisol (oh, hello again, my dear friend)—basically it screws with your body in many ways beyond just making you tired. But let's not just discount how *rotten* it feels to be tired from lack of sleep; it can ruin your day and affect your overall sense of well-being. That's why, when structuring an overall health program that includes exercise and nutrition, making sleep an equal priority is pivotal.

When I polled the members of my Facebook group about their biggest sleep disruptors, hot flashes and night sweats came out on top. The women in the group said they sometimes had trouble falling asleep, but even if they did drop off quickly they had frequent night wakings and couldn't fall back to sleep.

How can we stop this from happening?

HT, if you're a candidate, and sleeping pills from your medical team might be a consideration if you are chronically suffering from lack of sleep. But before you run off to the doctor, have you considered improving your sleep hygiene?

IMPROVING YOUR SLEEP HYGIENE

There are a number of things you can do to help make it easier for you to fall asleep and stay asleep. I have always had the sleepy gene but even I have had to change some of my habits around bedtime to ensure good-quality sleep. I even make my kids and husband do these!

Nap times
When fatigue wallops you in the face it really is hard not to take a nap. I consider myself a professional napper, having the ability to grab a healthy ten-minuter during the day when needed. But this might not work for everybody. In fact, if you're struggling with your sleep quality, you might want to consider ditching the afternoon naps (#sorry).

Reduce screen time
I am always shouting at my kids to get off their electronics before bed, and for good reason. The blue light from screens, including television and smartphones, can stimulate the brain so that it's more difficult to fall asleep. One Harvard study showed that blue light from electronics can disrupt your body's natural circadian rhythm and suppress the production of melatonin, which is the hormone that helps us fall asleep. So try to turn off all electronics in the house for at least an hour before bedtime and instead pick up a book for some relaxing reading.

Avoid booze, coffee, and late-night snacks
Try herbal tea or water to replace alcohol and late afternoon caffeine, as these have been associated with an increase in hot flashes and anxiety.

Nibbling on chips and chocolate before bed is also not going to do you any sleep favors, so to curb your appetite, think about increasing your protein intake at your last meal. It takes longer for the protein to digest and it therefore helps with satiety.

Adjust your room temperature
Your body's temperature is tied to your sleep cycle. It drops slightly toward the end of the day, as you get drowsy, and starts to rise again in the early morning. So setting an optimal room temperature is important for quality sleep as it aligns with your body's natural temperature dips. According to the National Sleep Foundation, an ideal temperature for your bedroom is sixty to sixty-seven degrees Fahrenheit. Especially postmenopause, I've found that my body is always running on the hot side, so if that's true for you, too, then you might want to take some time to create a cooler setting for sleep. This might include sheets manufactured with moisture-wicking properties to help keep you cool at night. There are also sleepwear companies that specialize in cool clothing for bedtime targeted to menopausal women, which I have personally not tried. Have a fan on in the room or open a window to keep the temperature down, and consider having a cool shower before bed.

Turn off the lights
Go to bed at a reasonable time. Studies show that we're getting less sleep than ever, with the average person getting six and a half hours each night, and that's likely to be self-induced. We get distracted by our Netflix binges and YouTube clips, and all of a sudden it's nearly midnight. That's not going to work for you, lady. Go to bed with the aim of getting your seven optimal hours minimum per night.

Take supplements
Some supplements have been shown to help somewhat with sleeping. I suggest experimenting to see what works for you, and if in doubt speak to your health care provider.

- *Melatonin.* Melatonin helps regulate your biological clock and can help you fall asleep more readily. Unfortunately, our levels of naturally produced melatonin decrease with age, but especially during perimenopause.

- *Valerian root.* This can be found in both tea and capsules, and studies have shown that it improved sleep quality for those with insomnia.

- *Tart cherry juice concentrate.* I first heard of this supplement in Stacy Sims's book, *Roar*. The supplement is high in melatonin and is also anti-inflammatory. A study confirmed that older people slept longer and better when taking it just before bed.

- *Magnesium.* This is a naturally calming mineral for the body and can help improve sleep quality, especially if you struggle with anxiety. It has also been shown to help reduce other menopause symptoms, such as hot flashes and mood swings. It can also help with bone density, cardiovascular health, and diabetes. It's a good all-round supplement to take.

Have sex!
If you're in the mood, have sex! It makes me sleepy!! (Shhh, don't tell the hubby.) Actually it's the prolactin, a hormone released after sex, that makes you relaxed.

HOW TO DEAL WITH STRESS AND PROBLEMS WITH SLEEP

Feeling overly stressed and trying to get a good night's sleep during menopause seems to be a constant battle. I have had so many conversations with women who are just exasperated. They feel like they have tried everything within their power to resolve their issues but to no avail. Try the hacks I have outlined in this chapter—give them a real shot—and remember, if all else fails, please go and see your health care provider.

STRESS

- Allow yourself to feel "good stress," which can come from accepting a new challenge, doing a short, intense workout, or doing something thrilling. It can also be helpful to think about acute stress as a challenge that strengthens you and helps you perform at your best.

- Engage in calming, de-stressing activities to prevent bad stress from taking over. Such activities include:
  > taking a relaxing walk (especially outside)
  > being out in nature
  > getting moderate sunshine
  > listening to relaxing music
  > practicing mindfulness and meditation
  > getting a massage
  > doing slow, controlled deep breathing

- › laughing

- › snuggling a loved one or pet

- › performing yoga or gentle mobility/stretching exercises

- › doing some gentle swimming

- › taking a bath or soaking in a hot tub

- › relaxing in a sauna

- › having sex, either with a partner or by yourself

- › engaging in physical, noncompetitive play

- › drinking green tea

- Establish a routine in your life, while allowing some flexibility. This can help decrease your overall stress level by creating order and introducing predictability.

- Schedule active rest days so that your body can rejuvenate and rebuild.

- Find an activity that allows you to recover without putting any undue stress on the body. Yoga, walking, cycling, and swimming are great examples of such activities.

- Get walking and remember NEAT. Focus on moving every day, outside of the workout window.

- Try to understand your limits for good and bad stress, be good to yourself, and recognize your capabilities and tolerances. If your body isn't fully recovered and you still feel exhausted, fatigued, or too sore from a work-out, that would be a great opportunity for an active rest day.

SLEEP

- Create the perfect, cool environment that is conducive to sleep.

- Set a time each night to go to bed and try to make that a routine.

- Aim for a minimum of seven hours a night.

- Prepare for sleep by relaxing, reading a book, taking a bath, or meditating.

- Try to minimize anything that will stimulate you before bed, including screens, caffeine, and alcohol.

- Stop the late-night food cravings by upping your protein intake. On those days when you do end up short on sleep, stay full and fight cravings by consuming a greater than usual amount of protein.

- Avoid taking naps in the late afternoon, which could disrupt your evening routine.

- Try supplements such as melatonin, magnesium, and valerian root just before bedtime.

Calming the eff down takes effort. Many of the women I come across in the fitness and health world are A-type personalities, like me, who only do life at high speed, so when they get hit with the menopause wrecking-ball, learning how to slow right down is very challenging. Menopause makes coping with stress more difficult. Your anxieties can be heightened and your ability to calm down can be compromised, so you need to introduce strategic measures to combat this. This shouldn't be seen as a sign of weakness or "giving in"; it's a strength to be able to recognize that these are new requirements for your life.

— 10 —

HOW TO THINK (SHIFT HAPPENS)

ETTING OLDER IS especially hard for women. We live in a society that values us for how we look, and so we are constantly trying to measure up to unrealistic beauty standards—it's depressing and downright insulting. Despite the number of "real women" campaigns I see, which I adore, women of our age are just not represented or supported, and that puts more pressure on us to try to live up to outdated expectations. This rampant sexism and ageism is a curse, and I don't buy into it. Popular media has a lot to answer for, and it's my aim to get you to move away from anything in your life that does not represent how you feel or how you value yourself and your life.

Yes, menopause makes our skin less elastic, fattens our bellies, and dries up our vaginas. And yes, all of these things are difficult to deal with at the same time. But by changing the narrative and deciding right now that you are practically perfect in every way (that's my Mary Poppins impression), you can start to embrace what is happening to you and learn to love yourself again. So many women tell me they're just completely down on themselves. I fully understand that, but it makes me feel very sad, and I want it to change.

I've been there. Those extra crow's feet aren't my favorite, my slightly puffy belly wasn't on my wish list, and embracing those extra gray hairs hasn't been easy for me. Yet I look at myself and feel a new sense of calm and lightness. Yes, I'm getting older, but for feck's sake, I'm nearly fifty and I think I look amazing. And I feel this way because I've spent time enjoying the new me and focusing on all of my positive attributes.

These attributes are both physical and emotional. Now when I look at those crow's feet, I see years of laughter and stories. And I still have a twinkle in my eye, which means I'm still full of terrible mischief of one sort or another. My gray hairs signify wisdom gained. Nobody else looks at me and judges me because I'm aging, so why should I judge myself so harshly? Why should any of us? It's time that shit stopped. Stop comparing yourself to others and start focusing on your unique talents and beauty.

Aging is not lost youth but a new
stage of opportunity and strength.

BETTY FRIEDAN

PRACTICING MINDFULNESS

Although we certainly can't "turn back time," as Cher wishes she could, we can definitely slow it down. How do we do this? It's all about life's greatest gift, also known as the present. By being present in the here and now, bringing your full awareness to the current moment rather than focusing on the past or the future, you experience that whole moment, not just part of it. Being present slows down your mind, engages the part of the brain involved in executive functioning, and enables you to make more conscious, thoughtful decisions about how you can fully live your life.

I often regret not being as present with my second son as I was with my older boy. I remember almost everything about my firstborn. I thoroughly enjoyed every one of his firsts and can remember them to this day, because I was fully present in the moment. When I had my second son, life was more hectic and the days seemed too crazy. I feel like I blinked and suddenly he was four years old. I wish I had slowed down and just enjoyed that time for what it was rather than fussing to get the house cleaned or the laundry done. Life is so precious that we have to enjoy it right now.

We talked about mindfulness in Chapter 9 as a way to reduce stress; let's look at it again now as a way to simply *be*. For some of you it may already be a regular practice, but others may feel like you just don't get it or that you're bad at it; or it might seem exotic or completely out of reach. But mindfulness is really an easy practice to learn and can look different for each of us (remember, for me it's simply about being still with my thoughts and my coffee). Anybody can do it, and everybody can benefit from it.

Some people adopt a daily mindfulness meditation practice, which is something like going to the gym for your mind. Although the brain is an organ, it's often referred to as a muscle because it's so adaptable, and we can do exercises to make those adaptations happen.

There is substantial scientific evidence in the form of MRI brain scans that show how mindfulness can shrink the area in your brain responsible for stress and so can be beneficial to you if you struggle with high cortisol or anxiety. It also stimulates executive functioning in your prefrontal cortex; studies have shown an improvement in attention, working memory, emotion/mood, and impulse control. This neurobiological effect allows you to slow down, be kind to yourself, and live your life with more intention. Simplified, that means working in a mindful way helps you have more control over your emotions and be more organized and in control.

If you truly get in touch with a piece of carrot, you get in touch with the soil, the rain, the sunshine. You get in touch with Mother Earth and eating in such a way, you feel in touch with true life, your roots, and that is meditation. If we chew every morsel of our food in that way we become grateful, and when you are grateful, you are happy.

THICH NHAT HANH

IDENTIFYING YOUR VALUES

Values are the way you want to live your life based on what's important to you. Your values are essentially your purpose, and it's vital that you make choices based on those values. When you live your life to match your values, you tend to be happy and fulfilled. But when the things you do and the way you behave do not reflect these values, it can leave you feeling very unhappy.

Values are not the same as goals. Goals tend to be focused on a future achievement, such as losing ten pounds in six weeks. Your values don't have to have an end goal or destination; they provide a direction and guide you in the present. Mindfully living in the present can help you be true to your values and therefore yourself.

Identifying your values can be tricky, and they will probably change as you grow through life. The values I held as a twenty-year-old are completely different from the ones I hold now as a middle-aged woman. What is important to you right now? What matters to you that helps you get through life with purpose and integrity?

I used a test at ValuesCentre.com to identify my top ten values. From those ten values I then identified my top five by asking myself if I was proud of these values, if I could live by them, if I would support these values fully even if they put me in the minority, and if I would openly share these values with others. The answer to the last question is a big yes, so here they are:

- *People:* Having meaningful, close relationships and time to spend with the people I care about

- *Passion:* Living with a passionate and upbeat, fun-loving approach to life

- *Nurture:* Showing a strong sense of caring and feeling empathy for others

- *Health:* Prioritizing my physical and mental well-being and trying to stay in as good a condition as possible

- *Excitement:* Seeking opportunities to constantly develop and learn from my experiences

I use this list to check in with myself and ensure that I'm being true to these values and haven't gone astray. If things aren't going right in my life and I lose direction, this list is really good at pulling me back to the present and putting a smile back on my face. This has been a great way for me to make some pivotal work decisions, rather than jumping at every opportunity thrown my way, as is my nature. It has helped me take stock and be present to determine whether an opportunity really fits my values and therefore my family life. It has given me the opportunity to say no!

NOTICING AND NAMING

A strategy I love to use with my clients (especially those going through menopause) is "notice and name." It's a gem of a tool that I learned from my nutrition and coaching school, Precision Nutrition. When you have a behavior or a nagging doubt that doesn't support your beliefs or goals, you acknowledge that feeling by naming it. Nothing more than that. By naming that thought or feeling, you move it to your consciousness rather than stuffing it in a box to ignore.

Noticing is stepping back from an emotion or experience and observing it. Using nutrition as an example, let's say you think you're hungry and you reach for a piece of cake, probably from habit. Rather than eat the cake, you ask yourself if you're really hungry or if you're reaching for that cake because it's 2:00 PM and you're bored?

Naming is simply identifying what caused the emotion or experience. Was it boredom, real hunger, or habit? Naming the emotion is usually enough to stop you from eating the cake you never needed in the first place and to make a rational food choice! In this way you take control of your emotional brain and use your rational brain instead. This is a way for you to have control over your behavior, and it can help you in your decision-making process. Bad decisions often come from emotions, and they are usually not very rational. Pausing to notice and name allows you to be more rational in your choices.

This strategy is also effective in a stressful situation, such as when I'm in danger of snapping at my kids, which I hate doing. If they're truly pissing me off, rather than my knee-jerk screeching, I will pause, acknowledge (to myself) that I'm annoyed with them, and then react in a more rational manner. Life is so much better for everybody in my household when I stay calm in the moment rather than fly off the handle.

"Notice and name" can also be very effective in dealing with anxiety, which is prevalent in menopause and can be debilitating. An example of how you can use this strategy when you feel anxious is to acknowledge your anxiety by saying, "Oh, hello, anxiety," or, when big, bad emotions hit you, you could simply say, "sad." You've acknowledged it. It can help to put your hand on your heart and offer yourself some gentle comfort by saying, "This is hard, I feel sad, and that's okay." Or, "You've got this!"

Anxiety is terrifying, but it's not dangerous; it won't kill you. Try not to fear the fear or be sad about the sadness—just let it wash over you and pass. It is also really important to know that your feelings are real and worthy of being acknowledged. Using "notice and name" can help you gain some control over them.

COGNITIVE BEHAVIORAL THERAPY (CBT)

Another useful strategy is cognitive behavioral therapy (CBT), which is a form of talk therapy, which you would do with a psychotherapist in a structured way, usually for a short term. The therapy focuses on helping you develop strategies for improving emotional regulation and can help if you struggle with anxiety, depression, or other stressful challenges. It offers a systematic way of becoming aware of negative thoughts and feelings that influence your behavior. The best way to become aware of these thoughts and feelings is to be in the here and now and to recognize how detrimental your negative thoughts and feelings can be—and that they're especially unhelpful when they're about the past or the future, because you have no control over either. As I mentioned before, my oldest son spent some time with a CBT therapist, and it provided him with two significant takeaways. First, he learned to reframe stressful situations by learning more beneficial ways to think and behave, giving him some control over his circumstances. Second, he learned breathing techniques to calm his nervous system and reduce the element of anxiety that clouded the situation. Both techniques have improved his life, and I have found that adopting some of these approaches into my life, especially in peri-menopause, has been an integral part of my growth. CBT says that depression is past-focused, and anxiety is future-focused, so the best way to cope with depression and anxiety is to come into the present and be kind to yourself.

COMMUNITY SUPPORT

I also recommend taking time to find a community support network. Menopause is very isolating. I often have felt alone with my symptoms, especially when it has affected my mental health. When we're feeling isolated it can be hard to reach out for help, but calling a friend or finding a supportive community, either online or in person, can be a huge lifeline. Remember, you are not alone, and there is nothing wrong with you. We are all imperfect, vulnerable human beings just trying to get through the day.

Kristin Neff, a psychologist and researcher of mind-fulness and self-compassion, says that suffering and the experience of personal inadequacy are a part of all human experiences. By recognizing that we are not alone in our suffering (especially during menopause), it becomes a lot less painful and isolating. I am a huge believer in the power of community—in fact, I've built my business around it. The adage "a problem shared is a problem halved" holds weight, and if you are involved in a community, you can live forever—that's science, bitches! Well, okay, maybe not forever, but research has shown that being involved in a community can have a significant impact on longev-ity. "Good, close relationships appear to buffer us from the problems of getting old," says Dr. Robert Waldinger, a psychiatrist with the Harvard-affiliated Massachusetts General Hospital.

Using the power of being in the present, you can learn to love who you are, right now.

Truly embrace what is happening around you—the good, the bad, and the ugly—right now.

By accepting what is happening in your life and knowing that menopause can be challenging, you can give yourself permission to show yourself some kindness and compassion. Right now.

That's how shift happens.

BUILDING RESILIENCE

You may have heard this one before...

An old Cherokee was teaching his grandson about life.

"A fight is going on inside me," he said to the boy. "It is a terrible fight and it is between two wolves. One is evil: he is anger, envy, sorrow, regret, greed, arrogance, self-pity, guilt, resentment, inferiority, lies, false pride, superiority, and ego."

He continued. "The other is good: he is joy, peace, love, hope, serenity, humility, kindness, benevolence, empathy, generosity, truth, compassion, and faith. The same fight is going on inside you—and inside every other person, too."

The grandson thought about it for a minute and then asked his grandfather, "Which wolf will win?"

The old Cherokee replied, "The one you feed."

LIFE IS ALL about learning to feed the good wolf, and two important factors in building the resilience you need to make it through menopause are being kind to yourself and knowing your strengths.

When you've had an angry outburst or an explosive argument, do you punish yourself afterward? It's pretty common to beat ourselves up, yet doing the exact opposite and showing yourself some kindness instead will get you back on track much faster.

When you develop a friendship with yourself you can provide yourself with support and compassion in your angriest, most anxious, and saddest states. When we are agitated and in fight-or-flight mode, showing ourselves kindness helps us to re-center and regain our executive functioning and the ability to be mindful about what we say, what we do, and how we cope with difficulty and conflict. If we accept our negative emotions rather than fighting them, we can keep them under control without denying that we are feeling them. Often, our most difficult emotions carry important messages about how we can make life better for ourselves. If we push them away, we miss the message.

And remember, showing compassion to yourself isn't about telling the negative, critical voice to "Shut up!" or "Eff off!" (no matter how much you might want to). It's about treating that voice with kindness and compassion, because, after all, that's you, too! Getting angry at the evil wolf feeds him more. Deep breathing, positive or compassionate self-talk, singing your favorite song, physically hugging yourself, and putting your hand on your heart are all great ways to soothe yourself. Sometimes that critical voice just needs a hug. Jump off the struggle bus and jump onto the snuggle bus.

If you're beating yourself up for eating cake, missing a workout, or yelling at your kids, give yourself a break. You're doing your best. You're only human, and life is hard and exhausting. You'll get back on the horse tomorrow. Don't get mad at that bitchy, critical voice—she just needs some love. Maybe it's the teenage you, still trying to fit in. I tell my clients to just chuck it in the fuck-it bucket. It really isn't worth your time and energy getting mad at yourself.

KNOWING YOUR STRENGTHS

You already know your values and your purpose in life, so as we come to the end of the book, what better thing to focus on than your strengths. Another great way to feed the good wolf is to know your strengths and build on them. When you've identified what you're good at, you can start to do daily things to build on these strengths. The research shows that identifying and then living by your strengths leads to overall improvement in your well-being, enhanced health, improved relationships, and a greater ability to manage and overcome problems.

You could start by making a list of the things you like about yourself, or, even better, take the strengths test at ViaCharacter.org. Character strengths are the qualities that come most naturally to you and help you to thrive in your life. This test is based on decades of research in positive psychology, which is the scientific study of what makes life worth living. Sometimes it's difficult for us to identify exactly what our own strengths are. These tests make that easier for you.

When I did the Via Character test, I discovered that one of my greatest strengths was curiosity. I was not expecting that at all. I assumed that one of my greatest strengths would be kindness or humor—both came up in the results—but yeah, curiosity beat them both. Curiosity is described by the Via Character test as "Taking an interest in ongoing experience for its own sake; finding fascinating subjects and topics; exploring and discovering." This is so true of me—after all, that's why I'm writing this book and continue to research the bejeezus out of menopause for y'all!

I do my best to put my top strengths into action. They look something like this:

- *Curiosity:* I read a book or article and share my findings with my followers. My favorite thing is to go down a rabbit hole searching for new information.

- *Kindness:* I try to sprinkle that shit everywhere!

- *Social intelligence* (being aware of the motives/feelings of others and of oneself; knowing what to do to fit into different social situations; knowing what makes other people tick): This one comes so naturally to me that I feel terrible if I ever offend anybody.

- *Humor:* I can be serious when I want to be, but I do like to see the lighter side of life and share that with others when I can.

- *Creativity:* This is a fun one to practice. You can find me most nights at home knitting, crocheting, making origami, or whipping up some baked goods. I get huge satisfaction out of creating something from scratch.

By working with my strengths, I give myself small wins each day. I create an environment where I'm going to be successful and happy, and therefore the people I surround myself with are going to benefit. Try it. I promise you it will vastly improve your life and help you thrive.

PULLING IT ALL TOGETHER

We are all works in progress. Life is a series of developmental phases. Your ability to be flexible, adapt, and build on your strengths will help you to continue making positive gains well into late adulthood. But in the same way that you prioritize and set goals for physical fitness and healthy eating, you need to do the same for your mental health. Physical and mental health go hand-in-hand.

If you had asked me five years ago if I had a mindfulness practice, if I had a value system, or if I worked with my strengths, I would have thrown you the stink-eye with my favorite resting bitch face in disbelief. I have never had to face physical or emotional challenges for such a sustained period of time as I have with menopause. The whole experience has completely changed me, and changed me for the better. It has given me the opportunity to really understand what makes me tick and what is important in my life.

You can do the same. These tools have been both an eye-opener and a game-changer for me. They have helped me put things in perspective and set me on the right track. I no longer feel the despair I did five years ago, when life just seemed too hard and I felt past my prime. I now have a renewed zest for life that I'm determined not to lose.

Dr. Christiane Northrup, the menopause queen, says that a woman's life has two halves. The first half is spent caring for others (children, spouses, and parents); everybody else takes priority, and a woman has little time to take care of herself. In the second part of her life, after menopause, she has time to take care of herself and to do things that support her values, and she is more at peace.

This is your time, ladies. It's your opportunity to use all of the wisdom you have gained to create a new life for yourself that's full of adventure and opportunity. It's a time to try the things you've always wanted to try and to live a life that puts you in the driver's seat. You see that light at the end of the tunnel? That's your light, and I want you to rip off your sweaty bra and run toward it shouting at the top of your lungs, "What's next for me?" And then go forth and grab it!

(This chapter was co-authored with Allison McColl, registered psychotherapist with the College of Registered Psychotherapists of Ontario.)

Here's how!

- Take five minutes in the morning to do some mindful breathing. Try "box-breathing" from Chapter 4, trying to empty your mind of all thoughts and focus on your breath. Keep in mind that there are no mistakes in meditation.

- Notice and name your negative thoughts and behaviors and just let them go.

- Download a meditation app that offers guided meditations for a variety of activities. Some great ones are Headspace, Calm, and Clarity.

- Go for a mindful walk. Try to empty your mind and focus just on the sounds, sights, and sensations. Feel the breeze on your skin or notice the sun in the sky. Feel gratitude toward your body for how it moves and breathes.

- When you are mad, sad, or scared, offer yourself comfort. Take a deep breath and remind yourself of all the shit you've dealt with and survived in your lifetime. With gentle curiosity you can ask yourself, "Is this feeling trying to tell me something?"

- Make a list of the things you like about yourself, or times where you really shone. Ask your loved ones what they like or admire about you. Make a list and look at it when you're feeling down.

- Connect, connect, connect! Surround yourself with people who love you and see yourself through their eyes. Research suggests that the single most important factor in longevity is social connection.

- Identify your values and live your life being true to them. Visit ValuesCentre.com to discover your purpose.

- Discover your character strengths at ViaCharacter.org.

- Whenever you're faced with a problem that seems overwhelming and unsolvable, remember a time when you felt the same way and things worked out. What is different this time?

EPILOGUE

We're in this together.
If we think together and work together,
good things are going to happen.

BILL NYE

I HAVE GIVEN YOU a lot of information in this book, more than you can consume in one reading, so I suggest you keep picking it up and coming back to it. Reread certain chapters when you need to. Menopause symptoms peak and trough; each one of the hacks will be relevant to you at different phases of your menopause journey. You need to identify where you are in the process and focus on the hacks that make the most sense to you right now.

At the beginning of writing this book, I started to feel some of the unwelcome symptoms of menopause returning. A low-grade migraine started hanging around, and I could feel my own Eeyore dark cloud start to form over my head. A few personal situations left me reeling, and I realized I was starting to go back under in my depression. I felt like a piece of black silk was slowly enveloping my head, smothering me, and stopping me dead in my tracks. I had previously come off my antidepressants with the guidance of my doctor, but I realized right away that I needed to get back onto them. Immediately I felt a sense of shame and frustration. The tears wouldn't stop falling. Here I was again, the fitness professional telling everybody what to do during menopause but feeling like I was failing myself. I felt like an impostor, a fraud.

But there were positives during that time that are worth sharing. I immediately sat my husband down and told him what was happening. He was prepared and completely understanding; our lines of communication were open, and by sharing what was happening to me, I knew I could get well again.

The other thing that I took from that experience was the importance of being proactive. Experience, education, and being completely in tune with my body made me know that I did still have control. Yes, depression had returned—and, with that, fatigue and lack of drive—but my stress levels felt relatively good, my nutrition was on point, and I was still exercising, even if it was just moderately. I was still taking charge of all the other aspects of my life. That was a good feeling.

The strategies I share in this book are here to help ease you through menopause. Your body is built to handle it, but that journey isn't always easy and it's definitely not linear. Be patient with yourself and weather the new storms when they come along. Don't give in to them, and don't stop taking care of yourself.

Patience and kindness are two of my best friends right now. I am in a good place, and I know that menopause is serving up opportunities for me. My hope is that you find your way through menopause in the sanest and healthiest way possible so that you emerge as a formidable woman ready to take on the world. Menopause doesn't have to be a negative thing. It can be a transformative time of your life. I am right here with you all the way.

ACKNOWLEDGMENTS

THE PUSH TO put my ideas into a book came from the driving force of my writing coach, Jo Macdonald. Thank you for your guidance and your patience in helping me take my dream to first draft. It seemed to take me ages to find anybody who might be interested in reading my book about menopause and how it impacts millions of women each year, but when Sam Haywood of Transatlantic Agency came along, she agreed that this was essential information for all women, and I was thrilled when she offered to be my publishing agent. Amy Stuart, writer, has been so supportive: she provided insight into the whole publishing process and offered guidance that was invaluable to me.

Thank you to leading menopause experts Dr. Louise Newson and Dr. Heather Hirsch for their input and guidance on menopause treatments. Tammy Pennington, RD, thank you for making me feel uncomfortable and challenging my knowledge of nutrition. I learned so much more than I expected from our lengthy conversations.

To my mentor and inspiration, Georgie Fear, RD, CSSD, author of *Lean Habits for Lifelong Weight Loss*, your sane, scientific approach to fat loss and nutrition continues to inspire me and make me a better coach. I also am thankful to Precision Nutrition for my continuing education in nutrition. I had many long discussions with my friend Allison McColl about human behavior and psychology, whether that was for weight loss, body image, or resiliency as we age, and I am thankful for her contribution to the chapter "Shift Happens."

The team at Greystone Books have made my first venture into publication a joyful experience. Nancy Flight was a great editor to work with, as she was keenly interested in the subject matter and really prompted me to dig deeper in certain areas of the book. Thank you Jess Shulman, copy editor, for making my random thoughts flow with meaningful order, for laughing at my jokes, and for pointing out all my inconsistencies (there were many!).

Lastly, my husband, Stuart, and my boys, Cameron and Eilean (who wants 25 percent of the profits from this book)—you have all been so patient and supportive, through all my menopausal turmoil and through my writing process. Love you all.

REFERENCES

CHAPTER 1

Bradford, Alina. "What Is Estrogen?" LiveScience.com, May 2, 2017. https://www.livescience.com/38324-what-is-estrogen.html.

Copaken, Deborah. "Exploring the Link Between Menopause and Alzheimer's." Medium, May 30, 2019. https://medium.com/neurotrack/menopause-and-alzheimers-1c455f29fe16.

Franceschelli Hosterman, Jennifer. *The Truth About Menopause and Weight Gain.*" Obesity Action Coalition, Summer 2014. https://www.obesityaction.org/community/article-library/the-truth-about-menopause-and-weight-gain/.

Garrard, Cathy. "Testosterone and Women's Health." June 13, 2018. https://www.everydayhealth.com/testosterone/womens-health/.

Jackson, Gabrielle. "The Female Problem: How Male Bias in Medical Trials Ruined Women's Health." *Guardian*, November 13, 2019. https://www.theguardian.com/lifeandstyle/2019/nov/13/the-female-problem-male-bias-in-medical-trials.

LaMotte, Sandee. "Hot Flashes Connected to Heart Attacks and Cognitive Decline, Studies Say." CNN, September 24, 2019. https://www.cnn.com/2019/09/24/health/hot-flashes-link-to-heart-attack-stroke-wellness/index.html.

Menopause Now. "About Crashing Fatigue." June 25, 2019.
    https://www.menopausenow.com/fatigue/crashing-fatigue.

Mohamad, Nur-Vaizura et al. "A Concise Review of Testosterone
    and Bone Health." *Clinical Interventions in Aging* 11 (Septem-
    ber 22, 2016): 1317–1324. doi: 10.2147/CIA.S115472.

North American Menopause Society. "Changes in Hormone
    Levels." n.d. http://www.menopause.org/for-women/
    sexual-health-menopause-online/changes-at-midlife/
    changes-in-hormone-levels.

North American Menopause Society. "Genetics Play Strong Role
    in Determining Age of Menopause and Overall Longevity."
    Science Daily, June 12, 2019. https://www.sciencedaily.com/
    releases/2019/06/190612110127.htm.

Richard-Davis, Gloria A. "Obesity and Menopause: A Grow-
    ing Concern." NAMS Meno*Pause* blog, December 14, 2016.
    https://www.menopause.org/for-women/menopause-
    take-time-to-think-about-it/consumers/2016/12/14/
    obesity-and-menopause-a-growing-concern.

Santoro, Nanette et al. "Menopausal Symptoms and Their Man-
    agement." *Endocrinology and Metabolism Clinics of North
    America* 44, no. 3 (September 2015): 497–515. doi: 10.1016/
    j.ecl.2015.05.001.

Society for Endocrinology. "Progesterone." 2017. https://www.
    yourhormones.info/hormones/progesterone/.

University Health News. "High Cortisol Symptoms." Decem-
    ber 13, 2019. https://universityhealthnews.com/depression/
    how-to-recognize-high-cortisol-symptoms/.

CHAPTER 2

American College of Obstetricians and Gynecologists. "Com-
    pounded Bioidentical Menopausal Hormone Therapy."
    August 2012, reaffirmed 2018. https://www.acog.org/
    Clinical-Guidance-and-Publications/Committee-

Opinions/Committee-on-Gynecologic-Practice/
Compounded-Bioidentical-Menopausal-Hormone-Therapy.

Clark, James H. "A Critique of Women's Health Initiative Studies (2002–2006)." *Nuclear Receptor Signaling* 4 (October 30,
2006). doi: 10.1621/nrs.04023.

Das, Renita. "Menopause Unveils Itself as the Next Big Opportunity in Femtech." *Forbes*, July 24, 2019. https://www.forbes.
com/sites/reenitadas/2019/07/24/menopause-unveils-itself-
as-the-next-big-opportunity-in-femtech.

Gibbs, Terry M. "Breast Cancer Survivors & Hot Flash Treatments." North American Menopause Society, n.d. https://
www.menopause.org/for-women/menopauseflashes/
menopause-symptoms-and-treatments/breast-cancer-
survivors-hot-flash-treatments.

Griffin Kellicker, Patricia. "Menopause Treatment Options."
Everyday Health, October 13, 2008. https://www.everyday
health.com/womens-health/menopause-treatment.aspx.

Hall, Harriet. "Estrogen Matters." Science Based Medicine,
September 4, 2018. https://sciencebasedmedicine.org/
estrogen-matters/.

Harvard Health Publishing. "Bioidentical Hormones: Help
or hype?" May 1, 2018. https://www.health.harvard.edu/
womens-health/bioidentical-hormones-help-or-hype.

Laskey, Jen. "Menopause: Questions to Ask Your Doctor." Everyday Health, June 12, 2019. https://www.everydayhealth.com/
menopause/menopause-questions-to-ask-your-doctor.aspx.

Newson, Dr. Louise R. "Body Identical Hormones (Fact Sheet)."
My Menopause Doctor, June 2019. https://d2931px9t312xa.
cloudfront.net/menopausedoctor/files/information/453/
Fact%20Sheets%20-%20Body%20identical%20Hormones.
pdf.

North American Menopause Society. "The 2017 Hormone Therapy Position Statement of the North American Menopause
Society." *Menopause: The Journal of the North American*

Menopause Society 24, no. 7 (2017): 728–753. doi: 10.1097/
GME.0000000000000921.

Rossouw, J. E., G. L. Anderson, R. L. Prentice, A. Z. LaCroix, C.
Kooperberg, M. L. Stefanick, R. D. Jackson, S. A. Beresford,
B. V. Howard, K. C. Johnson, J. M. Kotchen, and J. Ockene.
"Risks and Benefits of Estrogen Plus Progestin in Healthy
Postmenopausal Women: Principal Results From the Wom-
en's Health Initiative Randomized Controlled Trial." *Journal
of the American Medical Association* 288, no. 3 (July 17, 2002):
321–333.

Wilk, Katarina. "Chapter 11: To Take or Not to Take…?" In *Perimenopower*, 115–128. (Jönköping, Sweden: Ehrlin Publishing,
2019).

Wolff, Jennifer. "What Doctors Don't Know About Menopause."
AARP, September 2018. https://www.aarp.org/health/
conditions-treatments/info-2018/menopause-symptoms-
doctors-relief-treatment.html.

Woodcock, Janet. "Statement on Improving Adverse Event
Reporting of Compounded Drugs to Protect Patients."
U.S. Food and Drug Administration, September 9, 2019.
https://www.fda.gov/news-events/press-announcements/
statement-improving-adverse-event-reporting-compounded-
drugs-protect-patients.

CHAPTER 3

Cleveland Clinic. "Caregiver Burnout." January 13, 2019. https://
my.clevelandclinic.org/health/diseases/9225-caregiving-
recognizing-burnout.

Ladycare USA. "Is There a Link Between Menopause and
Divorce?" March 2017. https://www.ladycareusa.com/
is-there-a-link-between-menopause-and-divorce/.

McCarthy, M. M. "Estrogen Modulation of Oxytocin and Its Relation to Behavior." *Advances in Experimental Medicine and
Biology* 395 (1995): 235–245.

National Alliance for Caregiving in collaboration with AARP. "Caregiving in the U.S.: Executive Summary." November 2009. http://www.caregiving.org/pdf/research/CaregivingUSAll AgesExecSum.pdf.

Psychology Today. "Oxytocin." n.d. https://www.psychology today.com/us/basics/oxytocin.

CHAPTER 4

Continence Foundation of Australia. "Pelvic Floor Muscles in Women." January 2014. https://www.continence.org.au/ pages/pelvic-floor-women.html.

Girls Gone Strong. "What's the Deal With Incontinence?" December 5, 2018. https://www.girlsgonestrong.com/blog/health/ whats-deal-incontinence/.

Gunter, Jen. *The Vagina Bible.* (Toronto: Penguin Random House, 2019).

Hoffman, Jan. "The Cure for UTIs? It's Not Cranberries." *New York Times,* October 27, 2016. https://www.nytimes. com/2016/10/28/health/cranberry-juice-uti.html.

Mayo Clinic. "Vaginal Atrophy." n.d. https://www.mayoclinic. org/diseases-conditions/vaginal-atrophy/symptoms-causes/ syc-20352288.

Mundell, Jessie. "How to Do a Kegel the Right Way." Girls Gone Strong. https://www.girlsgonestrong.com/blog/pregnancy/ pelvic-floor/how-to-do-a-kegel-the-right-way-2/.

North American Menopause Society. "Changes in the Vagina and Vulva." n.d. https://www.menopause.org/for-women/ sexual-health-menopause-online/changes-at-midlife/ changes-in-the-vagina-and-vulva.

Ricciotti, Hope. "'Not Again!'—When UTIs Won't Quit at Midlife." Harvard Health Publishing, September 25, 2015. https:// www.health.harvard.edu/blog/not-again-when-utis-wont- quit-at-midlife-201509258353.

Shah, Maitri et al. "Treatment of Vaginal Atrophy With Vaginal Estrogen Cream in Menopausal Indian Women." *Oman Medical Journal* 32, no. 1 (2017): 15–19. doi: 10.5001/omj.2017.03.

Streicher, Lauren. "Slip Sliding Away: Dr. Streicher's Guide to Eliminating Sandpaper Sex." n.d. https://www.drstreicher.com/dr-streicher-blog/2019/12/slip-sliding-away-your-guide-to-eliminating-sandpaper-sex.

van der Laak, J. A. et al. "The Effect of Replens on Vaginal Cytology in the Treatment of Postmenopausal Atrophy: Cytomorphology Versus Computerised Cytometry." *Journal of Clinical Pathology* 55, no. 6 (2002): 446–451. doi: 10.1136/jcp.55.6.446.

Young, Carolyn. "Ask the Expert: Advances in Gynecological Care After Menopause." Johns Hopkins Medicine, n.d. https://www.hopkinsmedicine.org/suburban_hospital/about_the_hospital/news_publications/ask_the_expert_archive100419/advances_gynecological_care_after_menopause.html.

CHAPTER 5

Aronson, Dina. "Cortisol—Its Role in Stress, Inflammation, and Indications for Diet Therapy." *Today's Dietician* 11, no. 11 (November 2009): 38.

Breus, Michael J. "8 Ways Menopause Can Affect Your Health and Sleep." *Psychology Today*, July 19, 2018, https://www.psychologytoday.com/us/blog/sleep-newzzz/201807/8-ways-menopause-can-affect-your-health-and-sleep.

Brissette, Christy. "What Are 'Hormone Diets'—and Can They Really Help You Lose Weight Quickly?" *Washington Post*, August 5, 2019. https://www.washingtonpost.com/lifestyle/wellness/what-are-hormone-diets--and-can-they-really-help-you-lose-weight-quickly/2019/08/02/19ce5ab4-9f51-11e9-b27f-ed2942f73d70_story.html.

Brown, L. M., and D. J. Clegg. "Central Effects of Estradiol in the Regulation of Food Intake, Body Weight, and Adiposity."

Journal of Steroid Biochemistry and Molecular Biology 122, no.
1–3 (2010): 65–73. doi: 10.1016/j.jsbmb.2009.12.005.

Gonzalez-Campoy, J. Michael. "Obesity in America: A Growing
Concern." EndocrineWeb, February 14, 2019. https://www.
endocrineweb.com/conditions/obesity/obesity-america-
growing-concern.

Gupte, Anisha A. et al. "Estrogen: An Emerging Regulator of
Insulin Action and Mitochondrial Function." *Journal of Diabetes Research* 2015: 916585. doi: 10.1155/2015/916585.

Medical News Today. "Cause and Treatment for Menopause
Bloating." October 2017. https://www.medicalnewstoday.
com/articles/319609.php.

CHAPTER 7

Hansen, Mette, and Michael Kjaer. "Influence of Sex and Estrogen on Musculotendinous Protein Turnover at Rest and After
Exercise." *Exercise and Sport Sciences Reviews* 42, no. 4 (October 2014): 183–192. doi: 10.1249/JES.0000000000000026.

Hurst, Y., and H. Fukuda, "Effects of Changes in Eating Speed
on Obesity in Patients With Diabetes: A Secondary Analysis
of Longitudinal Health Check-Up Data." *BMJ Open* 8 (2018):
e019589. doi: 10.1136/bmjopen-2017-019589.

McDonald, Lyle. *The Women's Book.* (Lyle McDonald, 2017)

North American Menopause Society. "Drink to Your Health at
Menopause, or Not?" n.d. https://www.menopause.org/for-
women/menopauseflashes/exercise-and-diet/drink-to-your-
health-at-menopause-or-not.

Pellegrini, M., V. Pallottini, R. Marin, and M. Marino. "Role
of the Sex Hormone Estrogen in the Prevention of Lipid
Disorder." *Current Medicinal Chemistry* 21, no. 24 (2014):
2734–2742.

Rosenbaum M., M. Nicolson, J. Hirsch, S. B. Heymsfield, D. Gal-
lagher, F. Chu, and R. L. Leibel. "Effects of Gender, Body
Composition, and Menopause on Plasma Concentrations of

Leptin." *Journal of Clinical Endocrinology and Metabolism* 81, no. 9 (September 1996): 3424–3427.

Ruszkowska, Barbara et al. "Assessment of Ghrelin and Leptin Receptor Levels in Postmenopausal Women Who Received Oral or Transdermal Menopausal Hormonal Therapy." *Journal of Zhejiang University Science B* 13, no. 1 (2012): 35–42. doi: 10.1631/jzus.B1100276.

Scarlata, Kate. "Digestive Wellness: The Link Between Aging and Digestive Disorders." *Today's Dietician* 17, no. 7 (2015): 12.

Society of Endocrinology. "Adipose Tissue." 2018. http://www.yourhormones.info/glands/adipose-tissue/.

Yamaji, Takayuki, Shinsuke Mikami, Hiroshi Kobatake, Koichi Tanaka, Yukihito Higashi, and Yasuki Kihara. "Abstract 20249: Slow Down, You Eat Too Fast: Fast Eating Associate With Obesity and Future Prevalence of Metabolic Syndrome." *AHA Journals* 136 (June 9, 2018): A20249.

CHAPTER 8

American College of Obstetricians and Gynecologists. "The Menopause Years." May 2015. https://www.acog.org/patient-resources/faqs/womens-health/the-menopause-years.

Berin, Emilia, Mats Hammar, Hanna Lindblom, Lotta Lindh-Åstrand, Marie Rubér, and Anna-Clara Spetz Holm. "Resistance Training for Hot Flushes in Postmenopausal Women: A Randomized Controlled Trial." *Maturitas* 126 (August 2019): 55–60.

Burd N. A., J. E. Tang, D. R. Moore, and S. M. Phillips. "Exercise Training and Protein Metabolism: Influences of Contraction, Protein Intake, and Sex-Based Differences." *Journal of Applied Physiology* 106, no. 5 (May 2009): 1692–1701. doi: 10.1152/japplphysiol.91351.2008.

International Osteoporosis Foundation. "Osteoporosis Facts and Statistics." n.d. https://www.iofbonehealth.org/facts-and-statistics/calcium-studies-map.

Kjaer, Michael. "Counteracting Sarcopenia in Post-menopausal Women: Do Hormones and Strength Training Accomplish the Task?" *Clinical Science* 101, no. 2 (June 2001): 171.

Madhavi, Konetigari. "To Study the Influence of Structural Exercise Protocol on Physical Activity in Perimenopausal Women." *International Journal of Physiotherapy* 1, no. 3 (2014): 152–157. doi: 10.15621/ijphy/2014/v1i3/53470.

Mishra, Nalini et al. "Exercise Beyond Menopause: Dos and Don'ts." *Journal of Mid-life Health* 2, no. 2 (2011): 51–56. doi: 10.4103/0976-7800.92524.

Office on Women's Health. "Menopause." U.S. Department of Health and Human Services. May 23, 2019. https://www.womenshealth.gov/menopause.

Robyn, M., and M. A. Stuhr. "Exercise Through Menopause." *ACSM's Health & Fitness Journal* 6, no. 4 (July/August 2002): 7–13.

Silver, Julie. "Power Training Provides Special Benefits for Muscles and Function." Harvard Health Publishing, April 22, 2013. https://www.health.harvard.edu/blog/power-training-provides-special-benefits-for-muscles-and-function-201304226097.

Sipla, S. "Body Composition and Muscle Performance During Menopause and Hormone Replacement Therapy." *Journal of Endocrinological Investigation* 26, no. 9 (September 2003): 893–901.

Smith, Gordon I. et al. "Testosterone and Progesterone, but Not Estradiol, Stimulate Muscle Protein Synthesis in Postmenopausal Women." *Journal of Clinical Endocrinology and Metabolism* 99, no. 1 (2014): 256–265. doi: 10.1210/jc.2013-2835.

Woods, Rosanne, Rebecca Hess, Carol Biddington, and Marc Federico. "Association of Lean Body Mass to Menopausal Symptoms: The Study of Women's Health Across the Nation." *Women's Midlife Health Journal* preprint (2019). doi: 10.21203/rs.2.21012/v1.

CHAPTER 9

Bent, Stephen et al. "Valerian for Sleep: A Systematic Review
and Meta-Analysis." *American Journal of Medicine* 119, no. 12
(2006): 1005–1012. doi: 10.1016/j.amjmed.2006.02.026.

Harvard Health Publishing. "Blue Light Has a Dark Side."
August 13, 2018. https://www.health.harvard.edu/staying-
healthy/blue-light-has-a-dark-side.

Hill E. E., E. Zack, C. Battaglini, M. Viru, A. Viru, and A. C. Hack-
ney. "Exercise and Circulating Cortisol Levels: The Intensity
Threshold Effect." *Journal of Endocrinological Investigation* 31,
no. 7 (July 2008): 587–591.

Kanaley, Jill A., Judy Y. Weltman, Karen S. Pieper, Arthur Weltman, and Mark L. Hartman. "Cortisol and Growth Hormone
Responses to Exercise at Different Times of Day." *Journal of
Clinical Endocrinology & Metabolism* 86, no. 6 (June 1, 2001):
2881–2889. doi: 10.1210/jcem.86.6.7566.

Mindful. "What Is Mindfulness?" October 8, 2014. https://www.
mindful.org/what-is-mindfulness/.

National Sleep Foundation. "Menopause and Sleep." n.d.
https://www.sleepfoundation.org/articles/menopause-
and-sleep.

Pigeon, Wilfred R. et al. "Effects of a Tart Cherry Juice Beverage
on the Sleep of Older Adults With Insomnia: A Plot Study."
Journal of Medicinal Food 13, no. 3 (2010): 579–583. doi:
10.1089/jmf.2009.0096.

Sims, Stacy, and Selene Yeager. *Roar.* (New York: Penguin
Random House, 2016).

CHAPTER 10

Harvard Health Publishing. "Can Relationships Boost Longevity
and Well-Being?" June 2017. https://www.health.harvard.
edu/mental-health/can-relationships-boost-longevity-
and-well-being.

Mind Tools. "What Are Your Values? Deciding What's Most
     Important in Life." n.d. https://www.mindtools.com/
     pages/article/newTED_85.htm.
O'Brien, Melli. "How to Live Your Truth: Identifying
     Your Values and Mastering Mindful Living." n.d. https://
     mrsmindfulness.com/how-to-live-your-truth-identifying-
     your-values-mastering-mindful-living/.

INDEX

Figures indicated by page numbers in italics

ABOUT THE AUTHOR

AMANDA THEBE is a force of nature for women who are experiencing menopause and want to feel healthy and fit in their forties and beyond. With over twenty years of experience in the fitness industry, she is a highly regarded expert on women's fitness and health.

A popular guest on podcasts and at online summits, Amanda brings refreshing humor and a no-nonsense approach to subjects usually shrouded in shame. Through her very frank articles, hilarious social media posts, and inspirational and entertaining talks, she continually inspires the loyal readers of her website, FitnChips.com.

Her exercise workouts and fitness tips have been featured on websites such as Shape, Prevention, Healthline, Global News Canada, Lifehacker, Breaking Muscle, and Girls Gone Strong, and she has been a master trainer for Ultimate Sandbag Training. Her adoring fans and clients have called her "a resilient bitch" and "an unstoppable inspiration," with one woman naming her "the over-forty guru to watch."